# The HMO Health Care Companion

# THE HMO HEALTH CARE COMPANION

## A Consumer's Guide to Managed Care Networks

### ALAN G. RAYMOND

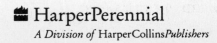

**HarperPerennial**
*A Division of* HarperCollins*Publishers*

FIRST EDITION

*Designed by C. Linda Dingler*

Library of Congress Cataloging-in-Publication Data

Raymond, Alan G., 1946-
  The HMO health care companion : a consumer's guide to managed care networks / Alan G. Raymond. — 1st ed.
    p.  cm.
  Includes index.
  ISBN 0-06-095080-3
  1. Health maintenance organizations—United States.
  2. Consumer education.  I. Title.
RA413.5.U5R39  1994
362.1'0425—dc20                                        94-29554

94 95 96 97 98 ❖/RRD 10 9 8 7 6 5 4 3 2 1

Dedicated to Alyssa Cyrene Raymond and Christopher Cecil Raymond, with the hope that they will grow up and grow old in a health care system that is compassionate, fair, rational, and affordable.

# Contents

# Acknowledgments

For their inspiration, guidance, and support, I am especially grateful to Charlotte Cecil Raymond, my literary agent and my wife of more than twenty-five years, and Janet Goldstein, my book's extraordinary editor. They helped shape the concept of this book from the beginning and kept me on track during its writing.

Ann B. Gordon provided invaluable research, writing, and editing assistance, especially for Chapter 7, "Making Your HMO Work for Your Good Health." Many of my Harvard Community Health Plan colleagues offered their expert knowledge and advice for that chapter, including Marc Bard, M.D., Rich Caplan, L.C.S.W., Joe Dorsey, M.D., Lois Estner, Anita Feins, M.D., Kathy Gardner, Joan Goldberg, M.D., Jim Harburger, M.D., Kathy Knight, Gene Lindsey, M.D., Dena McFadden, M.D., Annette Needle, Brian Orr, M.D., Sue Pauker, M.D., Alice Rothchild, M.D., Karen Smith, Sigrid Tischler, M.D., and Walter Torda, M.D. Thanks also to Todd Ringler and Leslie Solomon for their help with information gathering and to Betsy Thorpe of HarperCollins for her essential help with communications and logistics during the editorial process. And many others offered advice and encouragement along the way, which made the writing of this book a pleasure as well as a challenge.

# Introduction:
# Using the HMO Health
# Care Companion

*The HMO Health Care Companion* is for anyone who is considering joining an HMO or managed care network for the first time and for those of you who are already HMO members. It was written to help you sort out the myths about HMOs from the realities and to help you get the best possible care and coverage.

I've been an HMO member for twenty years, and I've spent more than a decade managing communications for a large and very popular health maintenance organization. During that time, I've found that there are two images that dominate the way people think about HMOs. Either

*HMOs have excellent, caring doctors, offer the best coverage imaginable, keep you healthy, and cost a lot less than traditional health insurance.*

or

*HMOs are impersonal and bureaucratic, they deny needed care in order to save money, and you can't even choose your own doctor.*

Not surprisingly, the truth lies somewhere in between. But where?

Numerous independent studies have found that HMO members are at least as satisfied as people covered by traditional health insurance and that the overall quality of HMO medical care is equal to that of non-HMO care. But as with any other service or product, not all HMOs are alike; some are better than others, and some are more likely to meet your needs and expectations than others. A successful HMO membership requires you to be an active participant in your own health care. If you make your health care decisions carefully and thoughtfully, before and after you join an HMO, you can maximize the quality of your health care and your overall satisfaction.

*The HMO Health Care Companion* is more than an instruction manual; you'll get one of those from your HMO. (Besides, as a top automobile executive was quoted as saying, "If you ever want to keep a secret from someone, put it in an instruction manual, because no one reads them anyway.") Instead, it will guide you through the decisions and choices you have to make; help you think about what is important to you and what questions you should ask; clarify what you can do to make your health plan work for you and what you should do when it doesn't work; involve you in maintaining and improving your own health; and help you get the medical care you need whether you have a routine medical problem or a catastrophic illness.

## WHAT YOU'LL FIND IN THIS BOOK

HMOs are more than just health insurance plans; they are health *care* plans. That's why you'll find as much here about how to get good care as how to get good coverage; with an HMO, they go hand in hand.

Chapter 1, "All About HMOs," is a primer for people who have never belonged to an HMO or who are choosing a new HMO. It will help you understand how HMOs and other

managed care network plans work, the advantages and disadvantages of different kinds of HMOs, and how they differ
from traditional health insurance plans.

In Chapter 2, "Making the Right Choice," you'll learn how
to gather information about cost, coverage, HMO networks
of doctors and hospitals, quality of care, and access to care,
all of which can help you to compare and choose among
HMOs. You'll be able to fill out simple questionnaires to
gain a better understanding of your personal health needs
and expectations and how likely it is that a particular HMO
can meet them.

Once you've made a decision to join an HMO, Chapter 3,
"Becoming an HMO Member," will guide you through the
application and enrollment process, describe who is eligible
for coverage through your membership, and outline the kind
of information you should expect from your HMO to get you
started. It also covers what you should do if you need care
right away, even before you've chosen an HMO doctor.

One of the most important relationships you'll have as an
HMO member is with your personal primary care doctor.
Chapter 4, "Your HMO Doctor," covers essential subjects like
the meaning of primary care in an HMO, how to choose the
best personal doctor, and how to develop a healthy partnership with your doctor and your HMO. You'll learn how to talk
with your doctor in a useful and constructive way; what to do
if you disagree with a suggested course of treatment; and how
you can plan for difficult health care decisions that could be
made on your behalf if you are too sick to make them yourself.

New HMO members—and long-time members as well—
seem to have the most trouble adjusting to HMO rules in
three areas: emergency care, referrals to specialists, and
"out-of-area" care when traveling away from home. Chapter
5, "Getting the  Care and Coverage You Need," walks you
step by step and question by question through these and
other important areas of HMO coverage, including hospital-

ization and home care. You'll learn how an HMO combines health care with health coverage and what that means to you as a member.

Chapter 5 will also help you understand a few of the essential fine points of your HMO member contract and how they may affect you during your membership, including benefit changes, loss of coverage, and coverage by more than one insurer.

Chapter 6, "Using a Point-of-Service Plan," is especially for members of so-called "point-of-service" HMO plans, which offer more choice and flexibility by allowing members to get their care provided and covered outside their HMO's network, at a higher cost.

HMOs don't just provide coverage, they organize and provide health care. So Chapter 7, "Making Your HMO Work for Your Good Health," focuses on how you can deal with a wide range of specific health care challenges you might face, including serious medical conditions, such as diabetes, cancer, AIDS, and asthma, or more common issues like maternity and women's health, pediatric and adolescent health, and senior health. You'll learn how to seek out the best care within your HMO; what questions to ask your doctors; and how to make your coverage work to your best advantage.

Chapter 8, "Problems and Complaints," will help you solve problems that can stand in the way of getting the care, coverage, or service you expect and deserve. You'll learn how to be an active and involved consumer, whether you are giving positive feedback, seeking a second opinion, or appealing a decision about your HMO coverage.

Throughout these chapters, you will find case examples, questions, and checklists to help explain how your HMO can work best for you.

Chapter 9, "Staying Healthy," contains recommended health screening and prevention guidelines for children and adults, and a guide to healthy behaviors.

In the back of the book, there are two other important sections. "A Glossary of Managed Care Terms" defines many of the common HMO and managed care terms you are likely to find in this book or in communications from your employer or health plan.

And finally, "Resources" lists some of the organizations and agencies that can help you get more information about HMOs or help you deal with serious problems or complaints.

With that introduction, get a pencil and some paper, and make this book, as the title says, your companion, as you choose an HMO that will be your partner in good health.

---

## About the Language of HMOs

In order for *The HMO Health Care Companion* to be useful for members or potential members of any HMO or similar managed care network plan, wherever it is located, the focus is primarily on the many things HMOs have in common. Unfortunately, one area where there are some differences is language. So you may find that, in some cases, an HMO you join will speak a slightly different language than what you'll find here. For example:

- An HMO member may also be called an enrollee or consumer.
- An HMO doctor may be referred to as a primary care physician, a plan doctor, or a participating physician, and medical professionals of all kinds may be called providers or clinicians.
- The document that legally defines your HMO benefits (what is covered and what is specifically not covered) may be called a member contract, subscriber agreement, benefits contract, service agreement, group contract, subscription agreement, certificate of coverage, or policy.
- The HMO department that handles member questions and complaints may be called member services, patient services, consumer relations, or member advisors.

- And then there is one of the more misunderstood terms in health care: "managed care." Managed care and HMOs used to be synonymous; today managed care is a very big umbrella that all kinds of health care plans and programs try to fit under. This book is about managed care provided by organized health plans that offer health care and coverage to their members primarily through selected networks of doctors, hospitals, and other health care professionals.

# 1

## All About HMOs:
## What They Are
## and How They Work

The kind of health plans we now call HMOs have been around for a long time. In 1929, the Los Angeles Department of Water and Power contracted with two physicians to provide and arrange all the medical and hospital care for two thousand employees and their families in exchange for a fixed amount per person (about $2 a month). Similar programs appeared in other parts of the country, organized around groups of doctors and clinics. Then came "medical cooperatives," which brought consumers into the decision-making process.

These plans were called "prepaid group practices," and they were fiercely opposed by many members of the medical establishment, who saw them as a threat to physician control over the profession. They spread very slowly until the early 1970s, when President Richard Nixon pushed through a federal law that created a new name for the plans, "health maintenance organizations," and sought to encourage their development as part of a national health care reform strategy. Nixon hoped that the thirty HMOs that existed in 1971 would grow to seventeen hundred by 1976. He and his advisors were more than a little optimistic; they vastly underestimated the amount of resistance to change that HMOs faced from the medical community and consumers.

In the 1980s, however, HMOs began to catch on, as they were organized in a variety of different ways to accommodate both the medical community and consumers. Their growth was also encouraged by employers, who saw HMOs and other forms of "managed care" as lower-cost alternatives to traditional health insurance. Today, almost one-sixth of the U.S. population is enrolled in health maintenance organizations, and HMOs can be found in all but a handful of states. Most HMOs are local plans, with their membership limited to people in certain geographical areas (their enrollment areas). However, there are a growing number of regional or national HMOs, and HMOs offered by large health insurance companies, which can be found in multiple states and different parts of the country.

## THE BASICS OF HMOs

Do you think doctors should be rewarded for keeping people healthy, returning them to good health, and doing so in the least expensive way possible? If your answer is "yes," then you understand what sets HMOs apart from other kinds of health insurance—their focus on prevention and primary care.

The health insurance plans that are familiar to most Americans pay doctors and other medical providers for each medical procedure they perform. Procedures performed in very expensive settings like hospitals and high-tech diagnostic facilities usually generate higher payments from insurance companies than those performed in outpatient clinics or primary care settings. So the emphasis is on sickness, not health; on doing more, not less.

HMOs and HMO doctors, on the other hand, benefit from

the good health of their patients. They are "prepaid" for the services they provide. This means that HMOs pay their doctors and other medical professionals an annual salary or a fixed amount of money per patient to provide health care to their enrolled members. HMOs and their physicians work within a budget, and they do better financially if they can keep their patients healthy, reduce their hospitalization and high-cost specialty care, and restore their health as quickly and inexpensively as possible.

Some people are concerned, of course, that if HMOs and their doctors are rewarded for keeping the medical care of their patients to a minimum, they might skimp on necessary tests and procedures; that in order to save money, they will withhold care or deliver poor quality care.

The challenge for HMOs is to find the right balance between doing too much and doing too little. Informed and involved HMO members can help make sure the balance tips in favor of high-quality, satisfying care that meets their needs.

## What Is an HMO?

Health maintenance organizations come in many varieties, but they share some common characteristics. In order to be called an HMO, a health plan must be able to provide and pay for comprehensive health care services to an enrolled group of members in a specific geographical area. Most HMO care is provided through a managed care network, made up of doctors, hospitals, and other medical professionals selected by the HMO to care for its members. If you are an HMO member, there are limitations on where you can get your care if you want it to be fully paid for by the HMO; you don't have complete "freedom of choice." With standard HMOs, care you receive outside of the HMO network will not be covered unless it is authorized or arranged by the HMO, or you have a serious, life-threatening medical emergency, or you are traveling away from home and cannot use the HMO network for urgently needed care. Some types of HMOs allow you to make your own arrangements for care outside the network and still be covered, but you will have to pay extra for that care. In brief, most HMOs work like this:

◆ You enroll in (become a member of) an HMO that covers the area where you live.

◆ The HMO provides you with a wide array of "medically necessary" services, ranging from routine and preventive health care to specialty medical care to hospitalization.

◆ It provides those services through an organized network of doctors, hospitals, and other health care providers that have been chosen by the HMO and that are affiliated with, or part of, the HMO.

◆ You are encouraged (or required) to choose a primary care doctor who will provide, arrange, or authorize the care you need. ("Primary care" refers to most preventive health care and to the medical diagnosis and treatment of most routine and common illnesses. HMO primary care doctors usually include pediatricians, internal medicine physicians, and family practitioners.)

◆ Every month, you pay a premium (or membership fee) that is fixed in advance, usually for a year at a time. If you belong to an HMO through the place where you work, your employer will probably pay part of your premium, and your share will be deducted from your paycheck.

◆ When you receive care from your HMO's network of providers, or when your care is arranged or authorized by your HMO, you usually pay very little (and sometimes nothing) extra for care; there are no deductibles, no coinsurance, and there is little or no paperwork for you to worry about.

◆ If you choose to receive medical services from providers who are not in the managed care network, you will have to pay for all or a large part of the cost of your care, unless it is a serious emergency or you are away from home.

◆ If you receive services that are not covered by the HMO's benefits, you will have to pay the entire cost of your care.

## Comparing HMOs with Traditional Health Insurance

If you have been covered by traditional (often called fee-for-service) health insurance, it is important to understand the differences between standard HMO plans and traditional coverage, starting with the basic fact that traditional health insurance plans pay for medical care but do not provide it. Here's a summary of the most important differences between HMOs and traditional health insurance:

| HMOs | TRADITIONAL INSURANCE |
|---|---|
| You receive care from the HMO's network of providers, and you are limited in your choice of doctors, hospitals, and other medical providers. | You make your own decisions about where to receive care, with few if any limitations on which doctors, hospitals, or other medical providers you can use. |
| You are covered for most routine and preventive care, as well as for the treatment of illness. | You are covered for the treatment of illness, but not for most routine or preventive care. |

| HMOs | TRADITIONAL INSURANCE |
|---|---|
| Specialty and hospital care must be authorized and arranged by your HMO or your HMO primary care physician. | There are few if any restrictions on how your specialty and hospital care is arranged, although advance notice to your insurer may be required. |
| There are no deductibles or large coinsurance payments, but you will usually pay visit fees or "copayments." | Coverage begins after you pay an annual deductible; after the deductible is reached, the insurer pays a fixed percent of doctor or hospital costs; you pay coinsurance. |
| There are no claim forms to fill out for care you receive inside your HMO's network. | You or your doctor must fill out a claim form for payment. |
| You pay all or a large part of the cost of care received outside the HMO network of doctors and hospitals, except in serious emergencies or when you are traveling. | Your insurer pays covered benefits for almost any doctor or hospital you choose, anywhere you are. |
| The plan is directly responsible for the quality of care members receive. | The insurer is not directly responsible for the quality of care members receive. |

## COMMON TYPES OF HMOs

HMOs have traditionally been classified by "model" types, based largely on how their physician networks are formed—according to whether an HMO's physicians are primarily salaried employees, members of group practices that have a contract with the HMO, or individual private practice doctors who have HMO contracts. The most common types of HMOs, and some of their advantages and disadvantages, are described in the next few pages. You may have to ask your employer or government sponsor or the HMO what model a particular HMO is, if it's not obvious from the way it is described in the HMO's marketing brochures.

These descriptions go only so far, however, since many HMOs combine one or more network types. So, while understanding the HMO models that are available to you is useful, it's only a first step in comparing, evaluating, and making an informed choice.

## Staff Model HMOs

Staff HMOs typically own and operate health centers or clinics, where the doctors and other medical professionals are salaried employees. A member chooses a personal doctor from among the health center's primary care doctors, who typically include internal medicine physicians for adults, pediatricians for children, or family practitioners for adults and children. Other on-site services may include obstetrics and gynecology, mental health, orthopedics, and other medical and surgical specialties. Staff model HMOs usually offer the added convenience of a laboratory, pharmacy, and x-ray equipment in the same building, and possibly some high-tech diagnostic machinery and an operating room for minor surgery that does not require a hospital stay. Some staff model HMOs own and operate their own hospitals; more often they have contracts with a limited number of hospitals that can meet nearly all of their members' medical and surgical inpatient needs.

Pros: Staff model HMOs offer the convenience of many services under one roof and there is the opportunity for coordination and continuity of care. In other words, when several doctors or other medical professionals are involved in a patient's treatment, they can talk with one another about the case and make sure that there is a smooth handoff from one specialty to another. It is also likely that all of the member's medical records are easily available to anyone involved in treatment, often on a computerized medical records system.

Staff model HMOs can also closely monitor quality and costs. When there's a problem with quality or service, they can directly bring about changes because they typically employ the plan's health professionals and administrative staff. They can carefully screen their doctors before they hire them, and periodically review their performance. And physicians who are paid a salary for all the care they provide, rather than a fee for each medical service they perform, have no economic incentive to perform or order unnecessary medical tests and procedures. At the same time, they don't directly profit from withholding necessary care.

Cons: Staff model HMOs offer a limited number of physicians at a limited number of locations, so if you join a staff model HMO for the first time, you will probably have to choose a new doctor for yourself and members of your family. (This won't be an issue if you are new to your community or choosing a personal doctor for the first time.) The fear that when you need care you will have to "take a number and wait in line" is no longer valid (if it ever was), but staff model HMOs can still seem bureaucratic. Most encourage their members to link up with personal primary care doctors, but patients can sometimes encounter frustrating delays when it comes to booking appointments or getting through on the phone. Staff model HMOs have been well aware of their problems in these areas, and many are focused on improving access for members.

## Group Model HMOs

Group model HMOs are typically made up of one or more physician group practices that are not owned by the HMO, but that operate as independent partnerships or professional corporations. These group practices may look a lot like the health centers of a staff model HMO, with primary care and specialty physicians all under one roof, or they may offer only primary care, referring their patients who need specialty care to physicians outside the group practice. Instead of employing the doctors and paying them salaries, the HMO contracts with the group practice to provide or arrange covered services for each HMO member who is a patient of the group.

Pros: Group model HMOs come with some of the same advantages as staff model HMOs: different types of primary care and specialty doctors practicing together, the opportunity for better communication and coordination of their patients' care, and an organized approach to improving the quality and efficiency of care. Some group model HMOs use doctors who participate in traditional insurance plans and in several different HMOs, so you may be able to join a group model HMO without changing your doctor. The group practices that participate in this type of HMO hire their own physicians and monitor their performance, and they have a direct interest in making sure that quality and patient satisfaction are maintained.

Cons: Like staff model HMOs, group HMOs may be somewhat limited in the number of doctors and hospitals in their networks, and large group practices have to work hard to avoid being too impersonal and bureaucratic. If the group's physicians take care of patients with many kinds of health insurance or HMO coverage, they are not as closely tied to a particular HMO as staff model physicians are, so there may be more variation in the way they practice, and the HMO may not be able to deal with service and quality problems as directly and quickly.

## Independent Practice Associations (IPAs)

The Independent Practice Association, or IPA, is now the fastest growing form of HMO in the United States. IPAs typically include large numbers of individual private practice physicians, who are paid a fee or a fixed amount per patient to take care of the IPA's members. Like staff and group HMOs, IPAs encourage their members to choose primary care doctors, who provide or arrange for most needed medical services and refer patients to specialists or hospitals when necessary.

Pros: IPAs usually have the largest number of primary care doctors to choose from. If you have a personal doctor and have been covered by traditional health insurance, you may be able to switch to an IPA-HMO without changing your doctor. If geographical convenience is important to you, you are more likely to be able to go to a doctor in your own community, or a nearby community, if you join an IPA rather than a group or staff HMO. For many consumers, an IPA may "feel" more like the traditional health insurance they are used to, except that the coverage is more complete and the costs are lower. Of course they also have to follow different rules than for traditional health insurance.

Cons: IPAs want to have a lot of doctors for consumers to choose from, so they may be less selective in contracting with doctors to be part of their networks. While joining an IPA may allow you to get your primary care from a doctor in or near your community, you will probably have to go to several different locations for other types of care, such as specialists and diagnostic testing. This means you may have to take more responsibility for coordinating your own care (within the IPA-HMO's rules, of course) than if you were a member of a group or staff HMO.

Since IPAs have less direct control over their physicians than staff or group HMOs, they tend to be somewhat more expensive to manage and it can be more difficult to monitor the quality of care their physicians provide. A resulting concern is that in order to control costs IPAs might impose overly restrictive rules on their doctors and patients, or place barriers in the way of needed care. Some IPAs have shown, however, that by linking their physicians through computer networks and by rewarding good performance, they have the potential to improve quality and efficiency in many of the same ways as other types of HMOs.

## Network or Mixed Model HMOs

Increasingly, the lines between the different types of HMOs are being blurred as they try to provide consumers with more convenience, geographical coverage, and choice of physicians. Many staff model HMOs also contract with independent medical groups; group models also include individual doctors; IPAs try to organize their physicians in "groups without walls." The advantage for consumers is more flexibility and choice; the possible disadvantage is that, while different kinds of HMOs have much in common in terms of their benefits, their rules for coverage, and their managed network of physicians and hospitals, there may be inconsistency within an HMO in the way care is provided.

Ultimately, it is less important for you as a consumer to understand exactly how the HMO puts its managed network together; it is much more important for you to understand how a specific plan might work for you.

## Point-of-Service (POS) Plans

When HMOs were created, and as they changed and developed over the years, there was one firm rule: If an HMO member received care from a doctor or hospital that was not part of the HMO's managed network, that care was not covered unless the HMO approved it in advance or unless it was a medical emergency. In other words, if the care was not approved or arranged by the HMO, you were responsible for the entire cost. By only covering "in-network care," HMOs could effectively manage their costs and offer consumers excellent benefits, preventive care, and low out-of-pocket expenses. But for some consumers and employers who were used to the freedom of choice offered by traditional health insurance plans, the "in-network" rules seemed too restrictive; they didn't offer enough choice. So a new option was developed, the point-of-service HMO, which is being used by an increasing number of employers to encourage their employees to opt for managed care network plans.

Point-of-service (POS) plans lie somewhere between standard HMOs and traditional health insurance in terms of benefits, coverage, and cost. They are not available from all HMOs or all employers. Any kind of HMO—staff, group, IPA, or mixed-model combination—can have a point-of-service option. When it is available, it may be offered alone, or as part of a "triple option" for employees, side by side with a standard HMO and a traditional insurance plan.

What the point-of-service option means, in the simplest terms, is that a member of a POS plan can choose to get care from doctors and hospitals inside the HMO network or outside the network, and be covered either way. If you choose to have your care provided by the HMO's managed network of doctors and hospitals, that care will be covered under the standard HMO benefits. You pay no deductibles and only small visit fees for "in-network care" as long as it is provided or arranged by your HMO primary care doctor. But unlike a standard HMO, the POS option permits you to choose a doctor or hospital that is not part of the HMO network, and still be covered. If you choose "non-network care," you will no longer have HMO-type coverage, and you will have to share the costs in much the same way as with traditional health insurance coverage. Typically that means you pay a deductible ranging from several hundred to a thousand dollars before your health plan pays anything at all, and you then pay from 20 percent to 50 percent (your coinsurance) for any care you choose to get outside the network.

Pros: If you like the broad coverage and low out-of-pocket

costs an HMO offers, but you have a favorite doctor you would hate to give up, you can pay extra to maintain that freedom of choice. You may have a child who has seen the same pediatrician since birth; you may not want to switch from the gynecologist with whom you have a long-standing relationship; you may want to have the option of going to a certain non-network hospital; or you may have heard that it is hard to get a quick appointment for a certain specialty with your HMO, so you would rather be able to find someone outside the network who can see you right away. A POS plan will cover those options; a standard HMO will not.

Cons: Most POS plans charge higher premiums than standard HMO coverage, and if you choose to get care outside the HMO's managed network, you will pay more in out-of-pocket costs as well. For out-of-network care, you will have to fill out claim forms and face some of the other complexities that come with traditional health insurance. You may also be responsible for bridging communication gaps that might exist between your HMO doctors and your non-HMO doctors if you want to make sure that your care is well-coordinated and that nothing falls through the cracks. Point-of-service plans are explained in much more detail in Chapter 6.

# OTHER TYPES OF MANAGED NETWORKS

In addition to the different types of HMO managed care networks described above, there are several non-HMO managed network plans that are quite popular. While they differ from HMOs in some important ways, they are also seen as alternatives to traditional health insurance.

## Preferred Provider Organizations (PPOs)

Preferred provider organizations are networks of doctors and hospitals created by insurance companies or employers to provide care at a lower cost than traditional insurance. About half of Americans who are covered by some form of managed care belong to PPOs. Typically, the insurer or employer negotiates a discounted rate of payment with the PPO doctors and hospitals and passes some of those savings on to patients. For instance, if you go to the PPO's doctors or hospitals, between 70 percent and 100 percent of your care will be paid for by the PPO; if you choose to get care outside the PPO network, you will be covered for only 60 to 70 percent. Since PPO care is less "managed" than HMO care, premiums are usually higher.

How does this differ from the point-of-service HMO option described above? There are at least three important differences: Many PPOs do not require you to have your "in-network" care coordinated by a primary care doctor in order for it to be covered. In-network care for a patient with PPO coverage is usually more expensive than a point-of-service HMO. And PPOs can impose restrictions, such as preexisting-condition exclusions and waiting periods, that most HMOs don't have.

## Exclusive Provider Organizations (EPOs)

Another variation in the alphabet soup of managed care networks is the exclusive provider organization. An EPO is usually made up of a group of physicians, one or more hospitals, and other providers who contract with an insurer, employer, or other sponsoring group to provide discounted medical services to enrollees. The arrangement is similar to a preferred provider organization, in that enrollees can get care without authorization from a primary care doctor. However, they must get their medical care from participating EPO providers exclusively in order to be covered.

## The Integrated Delivery System (IDS) and Physician-Hospital Organization (PHO)

Just to add to the potential confusion, you may also hear about integrated delivery systems and physician-hospital organizations. IDS and PHO both refer to networks of hospitals, primary care physicians, and specialists that join together to contract with an HMO or another kind of managed care organization, or an employer. They can make up all or part of an HMO's managed care network or they can affiliate with a different kind of managed care plan, such as a PPO or an EPO.

## WAYS YOU CAN JOIN AN HMO

HMOs are available in most parts of the country, but even in regions that have HMOs, they may not be available to everyone. There are several ways people can join; the most common is through an employer that decides to offer one or more HMOs to provide its employees' health benefits. Some HMOs, in some parts of the country, are also available directly, through a "nongroup" plan, or through Medicare or Medicaid. Finally, membership may be available through purchasing cooperatives or alliances, sponsored by government agencies or business associations. Here are some basic facts about each option.

### Group Coverage Through an Employer

HMO membership through an employer is usually referred to as "group coverage." Hundreds of thousands of employers of all sizes offer HMO membership as an option to their employees, usually alongside a standard health insurance plan of some kind, and perhaps with a non-HMO "managed care" plan as well. Some companies offer HMOs and other plans by agreement with a union "health and welfare trust fund." Small employers may offer HMO coverage through business associations and Chambers of Commerce. Many HMOs offer employers several options, with different premium levels, based on the makeup of the plan's benefits, copayments, and cost-containment features. It is not uncommon for employers to change their employees' HMO plans from time to time in order to control their health benefits costs.

There are two times you can choose to join an HMO through your employer: when you first go to work or become eligible for health benefits, or during your employer's annual "open enrollment," a period of time each year when employees have the opportunity to switch health care plans. A major advantage of joining an HMO through an employer is that most HMOs accept everyone who applies through their place of work, with few if any limitations on coverage for people who have preexisting illnesses.

Although an employer may allow its employees to choose from a list of several HMOs, it is not likely to offer all of the HMOs in a region. If you think HMO membership would be a good choice for you, or if you want your employer to offer a particular local HMO that is not presently available to you, talk to your personnel or human resources department or the person who handles health benefits for your employer.

## Nongroup Coverage

Many HMOs also allow people to join directly rather than through an employer. This type of membership is commonly referred to as either nongroup, individual, or direct-enrollment membership, and some HMOs give it a "brand name," like The Personal Plan.

Nongroup enrollment gets a little tricky, and it can be quite expensive because you pay the whole premium. Almost all HMOs offer "conversion" from group to nongroup membership. In other words, if you belong to an HMO through your employer and you lose your job, you can keep your HMO coverage by switching to a nongroup membership within a given period of time (usually sixty days) and paying the full premium directly to the HMO, either monthly or quarterly.

Some HMOs also offer nongroup membership to people who have not been enrolled through an employer. Chances are, if you want this kind of HMO membership, you will have to fill out a health questionnaire or take a physical examination, and if you have a serious medical condition, have been treated for one in the past, or are at high risk for illness, you may be rejected for membership. (Some states prohibit health screening and limitations on coverage for people with preexisting medical conditions.) Once you are accepted for HMO nongroup membership, you cannot lose that membership, whatever your state of health, as long as you keep paying your premiums and meet the other requirements of your HMO contract.

Unfortunately, since there is no employer sharing the costs with you, nongroup membership is unaffordable for many people. If you can afford to pay the whole premium, you will find that HMOs are usually less expensive than comparable non-HMO coverage. Unlike standard insurance, however, HMOs do not offer stripped-down "catastrophic coverage" plans for people who are willing to pay very high deductibles and coinsurance in order to keep their premiums lower.

For information on the nongroup options that might be available to you, call your state's insurance regulator (see "Resources" on page 241) or local HMOs and insurance companies.

## Purchasing Cooperatives or Alliances

Individuals and very small businesses have more trouble gaining access to affordable health care and coverage than larger employers. That's one of the reasons almost 15 percent of Americans are uninsured. One approach to solving the problems of access and affordability is to "pool" the purchasing power and the health risks of individuals and/or small businesses in purchasing cooperatives or alliances. These purchasing groups, formed either by state agencies or by business groups, such as Chambers of Commerce or business associations, often offer HMO coverage as an option, without the restrictions that can come with nongroup coverage. In most cases, the purchasing group will select the HMO or HMOs they will offer, just as large employers do. Consumers who join HMOs through cooperatives or alliances have to pay a substantial part of the premium, but they may receive subsidies from the government, or their employers may contribute part of the cost.

For more information about the availability of HMO coverage through cooperatives or alliances, check with your small business employer or your state's HMO regulator.

## Medicare

HMO coverage is also available to Medicare beneficiaries in many states. HMO plans expand or add to standard Medicare benefits in much the same way as the "Medigap" plans offered by Blue Cross and Blue Shield, the American Association of Retired Persons (AARP), and many private insurers. Most HMO Medicare plans include comprehensive coverage, including prescription drug benefits, with only a small fee for each visit. Just remember that you may not be able to get your care from the same doctors or hospitals or have your prescriptions filled at the same pharmacies you have used in the past. There are even a few HMOs that charge no additional premium for their supplemental coverage, but they will probably not cover prescription drugs.

HMO Medicare plans come in several varieties, depending primarily on how the federal government pays the HMO for its Medicare members, so it is especially important to understand the benefits and restrictions. Some will cover only care you receive from the HMO network of providers, except in special circumstances, such as emergencies and when you are temporarily away from home. These are commonly referred to as "lock-in" plans. Others will give you more flexibility to get care outside the HMO network; they work more like Medigap supplement plans. So some HMO plans will not work well for people who maintain winter and summer homes in different parts of the country or who spend much of the year traveling, because coverage is more limited when you are away from home.

Information on Medicare HMO plans is available from the federal Health Care Financing Administration (HCFA), which should have a regional office in your area; from your state's insurance regulator or elder affairs department; or from local HMOs.

## Medicaid

There is a growing trend among state Medicaid programs to encourage (and in some cases require) HMO enrollment. Medicaid is supposed to provide the poorest and most vulnerable in our society access to free medical care, but the program's costs have been rising out of control. Many Medicaid beneficiaries get much of their care in expensive hospital emergency rooms; they are less likely to have a personal primary care doctor who can help them with prevention or take care of common illnesses before they get serious. State governments, which run Medicaid and split the bill with the federal government, believe that HMO Medicaid programs can help slow runaway cost increases while improving access and quality.

The biggest change for someone who is covered by a Medicaid HMO or a "managed Medicaid" plan for the first time is that you will be required to get most of your care from an HMO primary care doctor and use the HMO's network of medical providers, rather than being able to get care from any provider who participates in the Medicaid program.

HMO coverage, where available, is free to Medicaid beneficiaries (except for visit fees in some states), but non-HMO coverage is also free, so why would someone with Medicaid benefits join an HMO voluntarily? Why should they play by the HMO's rules when Medicaid has no rules about where they can get their care? The reason Medicaid beneficiaries join, in most cases, is that HMO membership gives them better access to primary care and preventive medicine, and entitles them to the same level of care as any other person who joins that HMO. Some states also help Medicaid beneficiaries continue their HMO coverage if they get a job and lose their welfare benefits.

Information on HMO Medicaid membership is available from state and local welfare departments.

# 2

## Making the Right Choice: Finding a Plan That Meets Your Needs

If you understand some of the basics of HMOs—what they are; how they work; what varieties they come in; and how you can join—you already know more than most consumers do before they decide whether or not to join an HMO. But that's still not nearly enough. Before you can make an informed decision, you need to know what is important to you and your family, and how well a health plan can meet your most important needs. Then you can choose the plan that fits you best.

### UNDERSTANDING YOUR HEALTH NEEDS

Whether joining an HMO is your first choice or your only choice, you should be very clear in your own mind what you expect from your HMO. For example, the ability to choose from among many HMO doctors may be very important to some people, while others may be most concerned about being able to get care at a particular hospital if they are very sick. One person may be most concerned about a plan's mental health program, another about its preventive care for children. The questionnaire that follows will help you focus on *your* priorities by ranking some general categories that are of concern to most consumers.

In thinking about your own health care and coverage needs, or those of your family, rank the following from the most important (1) to the least important (6).

_____*Access to care*—such as the location of the plan's doctors and how long it takes to get an appointment.

_____*The benefits package*—such as whether mental health coverage, prescription drug coverage, or coverage for "alternative therapies" would be available.

_____*Medical quality*—such as carefully selected doctors and hospitals with high success rates for various medical procedures, and high patient satisfaction.

_____*Preventive care*—such as whether the plan makes a special effort to ensure that patients receive appropriate screening tests and immunizations for adults and children.

_____*Choice of doctors*—such as whether you can continue to use your own doctor and how easily you can choose a specialist or a hospital.

_____*Cost*—such as low premiums and low visit fees.

All of these areas are covered in detail later in this chapter, starting in each case with a brief "Health Needs Assessment" questionnaire to help you understand in more depth what is important to you and where you should focus your information gathering as you compare health plans.

# YOUR INFORMATION SOURCES

To examine or compare HMOs, you should gather facts from
as many sources as possible. Here are some of the places
you can find information about the HMOs that are available
to you.

◆ Employer, union health and welfare fund, or purchasing
group brochures comparing health plans (sometimes
called "summary plan descriptions"), and presentations
by your employer's human resources or personnel
department.

◆ HMO informational brochures. (You will probably find that
the information the HMO sends new members after they
join is more useful than preenrollment marketing material. Ask your employer or the HMO for a copy of their new
member guide and member contract. This written material
will also give you a sense of whether the HMO communicates clearly and thoroughly with its members.)

◆ The HMO's member service or consumer relations
department. (All HMOs have phone numbers you can
call for information. How easily you can get through and
how helpful they are will be another useful piece of
information as you make your choice.)

◆ Current or former members of the HMO.

◆ Your current doctor, if he or she has a contract with the
HMO.

◆ Your state's insurance, public health, or consumer
affairs regulators (see the "Resources" section beginning
on page 241).

◆ Business groups and health and consumer groups that
monitor and report on the performance of health plans.

◆ Consumer magazines that assess HMOs and other types of health plans, particularly if they are specific to your state or region and if they cover many aspects of HMO performance.

◆ For Medicare, the Health Care Financing Administration (HCFA) of the U.S. Department of Health and Human Services, organizations that advocate for older people and others with Medicare coverage, and those that monitor Medigap coverage.

◆ For Medicaid, your state's Medicaid program and organizations that advocate for people on Medicaid.

---

## HMO Advertising: Sorting Through the Claims

If you live in a part of the country where there is a lot of competition among HMOs and other kinds of health plans, you may find yourself bombarded with advertising campaigns on television and radio and in print, especially in the spring and fall, when major enrollment periods are taking place.

With the exception of the "feel-good" ads that some HMOs use (a single loon takes flight from a quiet lake as the sun sets brilliantly in the west . . . a family reunion brings together four generations of very healthy-looking people as the sun sets brilliantly in the west), most advertising focuses on one or more of the following themes:

Quality: "We provide high-quality care and service to our members; our doctors are the best; our hospitals are the best; our care is comprehensive and well-coordinated; we are rated the best."

Coverage: "We cover all of your medical needs; we offer 100 percent coverage; we cover routine and preventive care at little or no cost."

Cost: "We offer the most coverage for less; we have low out-of-pocket costs, with none of the deductibles and coinsurance of traditional health insurance."

Prevention: "We keep you healthy; we cover preventive care; we give you discounts at fitness clubs and in diet programs."

Simplicity: "We don't make you fill out all of the paperwork of traditional health insurance."

Physicians: "We have the most doctors in our network; you can join us without having to change your doctor; we choose our doctors very carefully and monitor their performance."

Location: "Our doctors are everywhere; we have clinics near you with all kinds of services conveniently located under one roof; we are part of your community."

Stability: "We have been around a long time; we are big; we are financially healthy."

Assuming that no one is guilty of false advertising (or that they couldn't get away with it for long), consumers are left to sort out these claims in much the same way they do for other products or services. Some of these claims may really set one HMO apart from its competitors, others could probably be made by any HMO. So you need to decide: Are they believable? Are they backed up by the facts? Do they matter to you personally?

Marketing brochures are a somewhat different story. While they are designed and written in a way that puts the best possible light on the HMO, they also contain useful information about what is important to the HMO, how it is set up, what kind of care is available and from whom, and what is covered or not covered. More and more employers provide their own company brochures that make side-by-side comparisons of key features for each of the plans they offer employees. In either case, marketing brochures can be one source of information in making your decision, but should never be your only source.

## WHAT YOU NEED TO KNOW ABOUT AN HMO BEFORE YOU JOIN

Choosing the right health plan can seem like an overwhelming task, but it won't be if you take a step-by-step approach to discovering what an HMO has to offer you. This section digs a little deeper into your personal health needs and expectations, and what you should look for as you examine an HMO. It starts with the six priority areas mentioned earlier in the chapter: cost, physician choice, quality, benefits, prevention, and access. The last section of the chapter covers some other important categories of information that can help you make your choice.

## YOUR HEALTH NEEDS ASSESSMENT: THE COST OF CARE AND COVERAGE

◆ If you have a choice between two health plans, and your first choice is more expensive, how much extra premium are you willing and able to pay each month for your first choice? $_____ per month extra.

◆ How many times do you think you and other members of your family will need to see the doctor each year?
(a) _____ Are visit fees for your first-choice HMO more expensive than others you can choose from, and if so, how much is the difference? (b) $_____
Multiply (a) times (b) to see how much more you might have to pay out of pocket for your first choice.
$_____

◆ If hospital and emergency fees for your first-choice plan are more, how much more are they per emergency or hospitalization? $_____

### The Cost of Care and Coverage

The biggest cost of HMO coverage for most consumers is the monthly premium. If you join through your employer, you may pay only part of the total premium; your employer will pay the rest. If you join directly (nongroup coverage), you will pay the entire premium, either monthly or quarterly. If you join through Medicare, you may pay a premium in addition to your payments to Medicare for Part B coverage (physician services). If you join through Medicaid, you will probably not pay a premium. Since premiums change from year to year (almost always going up) you will want to make sure that the HMO you choose is financially sound and has had fairly consistent premium increases. Otherwise, you may be surprised to find yourself faced with much higher than expected premium increases in the future.

Your premiums are only part of your costs. You will also be paying copayments (visit fees) for visits to your doctors' offices, for prescription drugs, and sometimes for emergency care and hospitalization. Most HMOs charge $2, $3, $5, or $10 for office visits and from zero to $50 for emergency care and hospitalization. If you are a frequent user of medical services, or you think you might be in future, you should compare these fees as well. You'll probably find that, even if your individual copayments are high, there will be an upper limit on the total amount of copayments you will have to pay in a year, especially for hospital care. You should also consider any special cost sharing your HMO requires for services like medical equipment or rehabilitation, if these apply to your situation.

It is important to compare costs, as much as possible, on an "apples to apples" basis for similar benefits or features. For instance, you may pay lower premiums for a plan that has higher visit fees or more limited benefits (no prescription drug coverage), or you may have to pay higher premiums and higher visit fees for an HMO that lets you use doctors outside the HMO network (a point-of-service HMO). So you should try to compare your total anticipated costs for premiums and out-of-pocket expenses, based on the worst case or most likely case for you and your family.

# YOUR HEALTH NEEDS ASSESSMENT: CHOICE OF DOCTOR

◆ Are you currently being treated for a serious or chronic medical condition? _____ For what condition? _____

Are you getting ongoing care from a particular specialist or hospital? _____

◆ Do you want to continue to see a doctor you now use, without paying extra? _____ What doctor or doctors do you want to continue to see? _____ Are they part of an HMO network? _____

◆ What specialists or hospitals would you want to be sent to for treatment of a serious medical problem? _____ _____

Are they part of an HMO network? _____ _____

◆ Do you want the HMO to give you information on the training and experience of their doctors? _____ What do you think is important? _____ _____

◆ If you are familiar with nurse practitioners and physician assistants, are there any kinds of care you would prefer to get from an NP or PA instead of a doctor, and if so, what are they? _____ _____

If there are types of care you would prefer not to get from an NP or PA, what are they? _____ _____

## Choice of Doctor

Consumers who are unfamiliar with HMOs may be concerned that they are impersonal organizations that are not interested in the relationship between patient and physician. So much has been made of physician "choice" that the reality of HMO care has been lost. In fact, most HMOs offer their members an excellent choice of physicians, encourage their members to choose a personal primary care doctor, give their members useful information to help them make that choice, and make it easy to change HMO doctors if things don't work out. You shouldn't assume you will have to find a new doctor if you join an HMO; your personal doctor may participate in one or more HMOs.

The place to start is the HMO's physician list, which should be available to you before you join. All HMOs will give you the names and locations of their doctors; some give you much more information, such as medical training and experience, special interests, and even photographs. This information can be very helpful in comparing HMOs, but it does not tell the whole story. A long list of doctors will not guarantee quality, nor will it guarantee easy access to care. Some HMOs have a lot of participating doctors simply because they are not very selective about whom they add to their network. Some of their doctors may be very popular and therefore have waiting lists for new patients; others may not have a long-term commitment to the HMO. If you see that a doctor you want is on the HMO's list, call and find out about his or her availability and involvement with the HMO.

### Is Your Current Doctor on the HMO List?

Generally, your primary care doctor is the only doctor you can receive care from without getting authorization or a referral. This means that if you want to see a non-primary care specialist, have medical tests, or need hospitalization, you must be referred by your primary care doctor. If the doctor you now get care from is on an HMO's primary care list, you should have no trouble maintaining your relationship. But before you choose that HMO, talk to your doctor. With a few key questions, you will have a much better understanding of how the HMO works and whether it will meet your needs. For instance, ask:

- ◆ Do you treat your HMO patients differently or the same as your non-HMO patients? If differently, how so?
- ◆ Is there anything you are doing for me now as a patient that you will not be able to do if I join the HMO? Is it important to my health?
- ◆ Does the HMO restrict the way you practice medicine in any ways that could be bad for my health?
- ◆ Will you be able to refer me to good specialists and hospitals if I join the HMO?

If any of your doctor's answers worry you, you should talk to the HMO's member service department or to your employer's health benefits department to get their perspective. It's possible that your doctor is misinformed; it's also possible for you to choose another doctor who has a different point of view. However, you are in for a rocky road if your doctor has negative opinions about the HMO or feels that his or her quality is being compromised by the HMO's rules.

If you cannot stick with your current primary care doctor, you will want to choose a new doctor. You'll find more on how to choose an HMO doctor in Chapter 4.

### How Does the HMO Select Its Doctors?

The way an HMO selects its doctors should be important to you. For instance, when HMOs hire their own doctors for their clinics or health centers, what general standards do they use? If they contract with doctors in the community, do they have a credentialing process? Do they require their physicians to be board certified or board eligible? Do they have screening processes that weed out bad doctors? Do they monitor their doctors' quality of care and the satisfaction of their patients? Do they have a way to discipline doctors who fail to meet their standards for quality and patient satisfaction? If an HMO's answer boils down to "We take any doctor who accepts our rate of payment," beware.

### How Are the HMO's Doctors Paid?

It is also important to understand the way an HMO pays its doctors, because of the common fear that some HMOs deny patients necessary medical care in order to save money. In general, HMO doctors are paid in one of three ways.

►They may be paid an annual salary by the HMO. Sometimes part of this salary is variable; in other words, they may get somewhat more or less money depending on how efficient or productive they are, how many patients they care for, how satisfied their patients are, or whether they meet certain standards for quality of care.

►They may be paid a fixed amount of money every month for each HMO member they are responsible for, whether or not they actually provide care to the patient. This is called "capitation" or "capitated payment."

►They may be paid a portion of their customary fee each time they see an HMO patient and have the rest held back until the end of the year, when the HMO distributes some or all of the money withheld according to how profitable it is.

Since the behavior of doctors, like the rest of us, can be influenced by financial incentives, it is useful to know what kind of incentives each of these types of payment can create. Ideally, financial incentives should be balanced in a way that encourages the HMO's doctors to practice prevention, perform all necessary procedures and tests, and recommend all necessary specialty and hospital care, but not provide or refer patients for unneeded care. Unneeded care not only drives up the cost of your care, it can be hazardous to your health. What is most important to you as a potential HMO member and patient is that your doctor applies the same high standards of care to all of his or her patients, no matter who is paying for the care, or how they are paying.

Here are some of the financial incentives that can result from the different ways your doctors are paid by HMOs:

*Salary:* In general, salaried physicians should have the best balance. They have no strong incentive to provide more care than needed or less care than needed. They could, however, have a bonus program that ties their pay to their individual performance. You want your physician's performance judged on quality of care and service, not just on how much money he or she saves the HMO.

*Capitation:* When individual doctors or groups of doctors are paid a fixed amount for each HMO member and then they are expected to provide and pay for all of the care those members need, they have a strong incentive to keep their patients as healthy as possible. Does this mean they will deny or withhold needed care so they can keep more money for themselves? You have to be convinced that the answer is no. If it is set up right, capitation can strike the proper balance between too much care and too little, but there is definitely a financial incentive to do less. The more an individual doctor profits by not ordering a test or procedure, the more wary the patient should be.

*Fee with holdback:* Doctors who are paid a fee for each procedure may have an incentive to do more, even if it is not necessary, in order to maximize their income. HMOs that pay their physicians this way tend to be more expensive than others. Since part of each physician's fee is held back, you want to know what the physician must do to get a bigger payout at the end of the year. Again, you want your doctor's year-end bonus to be based on quality and service, not just on cost savings.

Don't be afraid to ask an HMO doctor how he is paid by the HMO and whether the method of payment influences his judgment or his ability to practice in the way he thinks is in the best interests of his patients.

### Where Will You Get Specialty Care?

Another important part of your HMO's network will be its specialists. These are the doctors who will see you for medical problems that your primary care physician is not trained to take care of, and they can range from orthopedists to dermatologists to psychiatrists to cardiologists. If you have an ongoing medical problem that requires treatment by a specialist, you already know what your needs are. If not, you may have to see a specialist at some time in the future, and you want to make sure that high-quality care is available to you.

Some HMO health centers and group practices will have inhouse specialists: physicians who practice in the same building and who are readily available for consultations and referrals. Otherwise, the HMO will have contracts with specialists in private practice. If you have a relationship with a specialist and you would like to continue it, you will have to find out if the HMO will allow it and under what circumstances. For instance, even when a specialist you are seeing is part of the HMO network, you will need a referral from your HMO primary care doctor or the

HMO in order to be covered. If you have to change specialists in order to join the HMO, you will want to learn as
much as possible about who is available to you. Most
HMOs offer less information about the specialists in their
networks than about their primary care doctors, so you
will have to do some research on your own.

## Where Will You Get Hospital Care?

Although your chances of being hospitalized may be relatively small, you will want to know what hospitals are part
of the HMO's network and where you are most likely to be
hospitalized by your primary care physician if you need
inpatient care.

One of the hallmarks of care by HMOs is their ability to
reduce the number of days their members spend in the hospital. Many patients can and should enter the hospital "at
the last minute" before a medical or surgical procedure, and
should leave as soon as possible, not only to control costs
but to improve their recovery time. But that also means
that you want to make every day count in terms of the quality of care and service the hospital provides.

A second way HMOs control costs is by entering into
selective contracts with hospitals that are willing to give the
HMO a discount in exchange for a predictable number of
HMO patients. This means HMOs may only allow admissions of their members to those hospitals with which they
have contracts, except in special situations like emergencies
or for very specialized care.

There are several different ways hospitals are catego-
rized. Sometimes a distinction is made between "secondary"
and "tertiary" care in hospitals. Secondary care is more routine or elective care, such as childbirth, hernia repair, or
appendectomy. Tertiary care is more technical and intensive, such as organ transplantation or other surgery involv-
ing the brain, spinal column, heart, or lungs.

Hospitals can also be classified as "community hospitals" or "teaching hospitals" (also called academic medical centers). Community hospitals tend to be smaller, with a focus on secondary care, while teaching hospitals are the high-tech wonders where medical education and research are combined with secondary and tertiary patient care.

Some hospitals are best known for certain specialties, such as cardiac, maternity, or orthopedic care. And there are hospitals that treat only a particular condition or class of diseases, such as mental illness or cancer.

Before you choose an HMO, you'll want to know where you are likely to be hospitalized for routine medical and surgical care, including childbirth if that applies, for acute or high-tech care if that is needed, or for specialty treatment. While HMOs will provide you a list of the hospitals in their network, you need to make sure you understand which are actually available to you through the primary care physician, group practice, or health center you choose. If you decide that being able to go to a certain hospital is most important to you, you may want to base your choice of a primary care doctor on where the doctor will admit you if you need hospitalization. For instance, if you live in the suburbs but want to have access to a certain urban teaching hospital, you should try to choose an HMO and primary care doctor affiliated with that hospital.

## YOUR HEALTH NEEDS ASSESSMENT: QUALITY OF CARE

Check which of the following are very important to you in judging HMO quality.

◆ _____The HMO must have excellent doctors. How would you judge their quality? By their training? _____ Their reputation? _____ By how carefully they were selected by the HMO? _____ By whether they have access to certain specialists or hospitals? _____

◆ _____The HMO must have high success rates for various medical procedures. Which procedures? _____

_____

_____

◆ _____The HMO must have a formal program for measuring and improving quality of care.

◆ _____The HMO must be certified or accredited by an independent quality assurance organization.

◆ _____The HMO must receive high satisfaction ratings from its current members, when they are asked about quality of care.

## Quality of Care

Everyone wants high-quality health care. Independent assessments of the quality of health care rate overall HMO quality as equal to that of non-HMO care, but how can you tell whether the HMO you choose will meet that test? Until recently, there was a commonly accepted formula for health care quality: more is better. More services, more technology, more expensive care—all were thought to equal better quality. Medical experts now agree that's not so, and there are rapidly evolving new systems for measuring and reporting on health care quality, based on what is appropriate and effective. Let's take a look at two ways to judge quality in a health plan—the traditional view and a more current approach, where the emphasis is on continuous, measurable quality improvement.

| TRADITIONAL VIEW OF QUALITY | QUALITY IMPROVEMENT VIEW |
| --- | --- |
| More expensive, high-tech care is higher quality. | Appropriate and effective care is high quality. |
| More tests and procedures are higher quality. | High rates of preventive procedures and screening for disease mean higher quality. |
| A doctor or hospital with the best reputation is high quality. | Doctors and hospitals that meet measurable standards are high quality. |
| Freedom of choice of doctors means higher quality. | A choice from among doctors who are carefully selected and who work in close coordination with their peers means high quality. |
| A doctor I like is high quality. | High patient and physician satisfaction are elements of high quality. |
| Care that restores my health is high quality. | Care that keeps people healthy and that restores their health in measurable ways is of high quality (but reliable quality measurement is very difficult to do). |

Today, there is increasing attention being paid to measuring and reporting the quality of health plans, including the public reporting of comparable information that has been audited and verified by independent organizations. (So far, much more has been done to measure and report on the quality of managed-care health plans than fee-for-service health insurance, so it is difficult to compare the quality of HMOs versus traditional health insurance plans.)

The National Committee for Quality Assurance (NCQA) has been involved in HMO quality measurement and improvement for many years, and they recently began offering accreditation to health plans. Based in Washington, D.C., NCQA was originally part of the HMOs' national trade association, but it is now an independent organization. If an HMO has been fully accredited by NCQA, that means it has passed a rigorous review of its ability to provide, measure, and improve quality of care for its members.

But two warnings are in order. First, the measurement of health care quality is a very new science and apples-to-apples comparisons are still hard to come by. Second, quality is in many respects in the eye of the beholder. In other words, you probably have your own ideas about what high-quality health care means, and it may not be the same as how the experts define quality. An HMO that meets the needs that you've identified as most important to you will probably meet your test for quality, even if its quality scores aren't the highest.

## What Do "HMO Report Cards" Measure?

Another way to assess HMO quality is through the health care "report cards" that are being compiled and published by employers, government agencies, independent quality assurance organizations, and HMOs themselves. Most report card quality measures focus on the percentage of people who receive certain tests or treatments that are considered helpful in preventing disease or detecting and treating it at its early stages. These include:

◆ The percentage of children in the HMO who received all recommended immunizations before the age of two.

◆ The percentage of women receiving early and appropriate prenatal care.

◆ Pap-test screening rates for adult women (to detect cervical cancer or precancerous abnormalities).

◆ Cholesterol screening rates for adults.

◆ Mammography rates for women over age fifty (to detect breast disease, especially cancer).

◆ Yearly eye-exam rates for diabetics (to detect complications that can cause blindness).

With some measures, lower rates, either compared to other health plans or to national standards or "benchmarks," are indicators of higher quality. These include:

◆ The percentage of babies who are born with very low birth weights.

◆ The percentage of women who have their babies delivered by cesarean section.

Other measures focus on "outcomes," or how effective care has actually been in preventing medical problems or in restoring health. For instance:

◆ The rate that patients are readmitted to the hospital after certain kinds of procedures.

◆ The percentage of patients with certain types of cancer who survive at least five years after treatment.

A third category found in HMO report cards is patient satisfaction. Here you will find information on how satisfied an HMO's current members say they are, overall, with their HMO membership; with the quality of care they receive; with the way they are treated by the plan's doctors and staff; with the control they have over medical decisions; or with their ability to have easy access to care when they need it.

So how should you view consumer report cards comparing quality of HMOs? If it is based on independent, audited evaluations (rather than simply on the HMO's rating of itself), if the information is comparable from one plan to the next, and if it measures performance over time, a report card should be a very useful way for you to judge how well an HMO is able to maintain and improve quality. While some individual quality measures may not be important to you personally, an HMO that performs well in these measures is more likely to perform well in those that may have a direct impact on your health. Check with your employer about the availability of HMO report cards and ask for help in interpreting them.

## YOUR HEALTH NEEDS ASSESSMENT: THE BENEFITS PACKAGE

◆ Is it important that your HMO cover preventive care, such as routine immunizations and checkups for little or no extra cost? _____

◆ Is it important for your prescription drugs to be covered? _____ About how much do you spend each year on prescription drugs under your current health insurance? _____ About how often do you have prescriptions filled? _____ Where? _____ Does it matter what pharmacy you use as long as it offers good service and quality? _____

◆ Is it important to you for mental health and substance abuse care to be covered? If you are being treated, how often? _____ Does it matter what doctor you see or what program you are in as long as you get good care? _____

◆ Is it important to you for "alternative therapies" such as chiropractic, acupuncture, biofeedback, etc. to be covered? _____ Which do you use? _____

_____ How often do you use these
treatments? _____ Are you willing to pay
extra to continue? _____

## The Benefits Package

Certainly one of the most important questions you will
want answered is, Will my HMO cover the care I need? In
general, HMOs have very comprehensive benefits for routine and preventive care as well as treatment for serious illness, specialty care, and hospitalization. Benefit summary
charts are readily available from all HMOs and they're usually easy to compare. But they do not tell the whole story
unless they also tell you what is not covered (exclusions).
And even then, there may be gray areas where definitions
and coverage rules are anything but clear-cut.

Most HMOs cover what they call "medically necessary
care," including services, procedures, devices, or drugs that
are safe, appropriate, and effective for the prevention, evaluation, or treatment of medical conditions. However, they do
not cover everything that is medically beneficial; they may
not cover some types of care that _you_ think are appropriate
and effective, such as acupuncture or chiropractic; and they
will probably not cover treatment that is considered "experimental" or "unproven."

With medical technology advancing so rapidly, you would
be wise to understand how the HMO defines "experimental"
and how it decides when a particular form of treatment,
whether it is a new drug or a new form of surgery, is no
longer considered experimental. Most HMOs use strict guidelines, based on the results of controlled medical trials and the
endorsement or guidelines of federal government organizations, such as the U.S. Food and Drug Administration (FDA)
or professional medical organizations, to decide whether a

procedure is experimental. Some HMOs give their physicians a certain amount of leeway to make the medical decisions they think are best for their patients, even when they may involve experimental procedures.

---

### When Is a New Therapy Experimental?

The most difficult issues involve procedures that may be the last hope for a patient who is desperately ill. A recent example is a treatment for advanced breast cancer that requires high-dose chemotherapy and the replacement of destroyed bone marrow through a process called autologous bone marrow transplantation (ABMT). Some HMOs and insurance companies have argued that since there is no conclusive evidence that it is safe or any more effective than more conventional types of treatment, it should still be considered experimental. Supporters of the procedure say that it is the only hope for extending the life of women with advanced disease, and should therefore be covered. A compromise position that some HMOs and insurers have taken is to cover ABMT under certain circumstances or to try to get their members who qualify into clinical trials that would provide the treatment under controlled conditions and contribute to research on its effectiveness.

The medical, ethical, and financial issues involved in deciding where to "draw the line" are among the most difficult faced by our generation, not just for HMOs, but for all who provide or pay for health care. As an HMO member, you'll want to be sure that coverage decisions in these gray areas will not be based on cost alone. At the same time, you need to keep in mind that more is not always better in medical care; that not everything can or should be covered. Ask whether the HMO has a formal committee or process for assessing new technologies and deciding whether they should be made available and covered.

## Will There Be Limitations on Covered Benefits?

Like all insurance plans, HMOs put limits on certain kinds of covered treatment. For instance, there may be a limit on the number of visits for certain kinds of outpatient care provided by an HMO doctor or at an HMO facility, or the visit fee may increase as the number of treatments increases. There may be limits on certain kinds of inpatient services, such as rehabilitation or psychiatric hospitalization. There is seldom a limit on the total dollar value of the care HMOs will cover. If there is, you want to make sure it is very high, since a single hospitalization can run into hundreds of thousands of dollars.

## Will There Be Coverage for Your Ongoing Medical Needs?

If you have an ongoing condition that requires medical attention, you will want to be certain that you understand whether coverage is available from the HMO. For instance, you may find that coverage is excluded for chiropractic care, certain types of infertility services, certain dental and visual services, certain medical equipment, services for learning disabilities, blood and blood products, and so on. These kinds of exclusions are not limited to HMOs, but you can compare benefits to see if one plan will meet your needs better than another.

Coverage is not all that matters; you also want the best possible care. If you have ongoing medical needs you will want to ask whether the HMO has special programs for patients like you, either as part of the HMO itself or at hospitals that are affiliated with the HMO. For instance, some HMOs have special in-house programs for the treatment of asthma, cancer, diabetes, AIDS, mental illness, or substance abuse. You can find out in advance if you will be eligible to participate in these programs and how they would handle your care. (For more on dealing with specific medical conditions, see Chapter 7, "Making Your HMO Work for Your Good Health.")

## What About Prescription Drug Coverage?

Coverage for the cost of prescription drugs can save HMO members a lot of out-of-pocket money. Most employer-sponsored HMO plans include coverage for the cost of prescription drugs, as do many Medicaid and Medicare HMOs. If you are joining an HMO on a self-paying basis, check to see whether or not the HMO offers drug coverage to its non-group members.

As with other HMO benefits, there are some limitations on what is covered, and there are rules for members to follow. Most prescription drug plans cover medically necessary prescription drugs and, sometimes, medically necessary nonprescription drugs and medical supplies. If there is a particular prescription drug that you use regularly, you'll want to ask in advance if it is covered.

In order to control costs and encourage more consistent quality, some HMOs develop limited lists of recommended drugs, either generic or brand name, for different medical conditions. These are called "formularies." You may find that an HMO will limit coverage to the drugs on its formulary unless you have a condition for which there is no appropriate drug on their list. This could mean that you would have to switch from a drug that is familiar to you.

Along with what is covered, you need to understand the "how" of coverage. Most HMO prescription drug plans will cover only prescriptions filled at pharmacies that are part of the HMO network (their participating pharmacies). These may include pharmacies owned and operated by your HMO, selected community pharmacies, chain pharmacies, mail-order services, or a combination of all four. Before you join, you should check an HMO's list of approved pharmacies, to make sure at least one is convenient for you. (For more on prescription drug coverage, see Chapter 5, "Getting the Care and Coverage You Need.")

# YOUR HEALTH NEEDS ASSESSMENT: PREVENTIVE CARE

◆ Should your HMO offer health promotion programs to help members stay fit, lose weight, or stop smoking?

_____

◆ What kind of prevention is most important to you?

_____

_____

◆ Is it important for your HMO to encourage and remind you to make use of preventive services? _____

◆ Is it important for you to know the percent of children in the plan who are fully immunized, when they should be, against common childhood diseases? _____

◆ Is it important for you to know the percent of pregnant women in the plan who receive appropriate prenatal care early in their pregnancies? _____

◆ Is it important for you to know the percent of adults in the plan who have been screened for breast cancer (mammography), cervical cancer (Pap smears), colon cancer, high cholesterol, high blood pressure, and other serious diseases? _____ Which screening tests are most important to you? _____

_____

## Preventive Care

There's no question that avoiding an illness or catching it in its earliest stages is better for the patient, and generally less expensive, than having to treat it after it becomes more serious. An ounce of prevention really is worth a pound of cure. The most effective preventive care will occur if you, your HMO doctor, and your HMO all take an active role. Prevention can be divided into three broad categories:

◆ Those things that will actually prevent disease or other medical problems in the first place. Some of the best examples are immunizations for you and your children and certain types of prenatal care, and, of course, changing your own behavior to reduce the risk of illness or accident. (The U. S. government's Preventive Services Task Force has stated that "the most promising role for prevention in current medical practice may lie in changing the personal health behaviors of patients long before clinical disease develops.")

◆ Those things that will help detect disease or the risk of disease at its early stages so that treatment can be more effective. These include cholesterol screening, blood pressure testing, Pap smears, mammography screening, and rectal, breast, and testicular examinations.

◆ Those things that help patients avoid medical crises and emergency hospitalization by carefully managing, or helping them manage, their ongoing care for diseases like asthma, diabetes, or high blood pressure.

Many people have been attracted to HMOs because they have always covered preventive practices, like vaccinations, prenatal care, and screening tests, while traditional health insurance plans have not. The trend today is for HMOs to develop standard guidelines for the kinds of preventive care they recommend for their members of different ages. (You'll find a complete set of guidelines in Chapter 9, "Staying Healthy.") Some HMOs will cover only preventive care that falls within their guidelines. For instance, an HMO may cover certain tests only if they are conducted at recommended intervals, unless you are considered at high risk for a certain disease. This information should be spelled out in the HMO's member contract.

Another consideration, which may not be as obvious in the contract, is whether there are some tests an HMO does not cover. Some preventive measures may be considered experimental, not cost effective, or unproven. Examples include certain types of nutritional or vitamin therapies, "preventive" chiropractic care, and biofeedback. You may swear by them, but HMOs may exclude or limit their coverage because they are not considered medically necessary or proven effective.

Check the exclusions section of the HMO member contract and ask the HMO's member service department, if you have questions about coverage of a specific type of preventive care. Here are some key issues to consider:

◆ Does the HMO have standards for the appropriate frequency of preventive tests, and if so, are they simply guidelines or are they rules you would have to follow in order to be covered?

◆ Are there any restrictions on who can perform routine exams? For instance, if you are a woman, can you go to a gynecologist for routine gynecological services or do they have to be performed or authorized by your primary care doctor?

◆ Does the HMO remind members when well-baby care or a vaccination or preventive test is due?

◆ Are physicals for school, camp, jobs, job training, certification, or life insurance covered, or are they covered only when they can be done during a scheduled routine physical?

◆ What programs or classes does the HMO offer to help you change unhealthy behaviors such as smoking, deal with problems like weight management and stress, or manage medical conditions like asthma, diabetes, or back pain?

◆ For a screening test or other type of preventive care not covered by the HMO, could you ask your HMO doctor to perform it and pay for it yourself?

## YOUR HEALTH NEEDS ASSESSMENT: ACCESS TO CARE

◆ How far are you willing to travel to see your personal, primary care doctor? _____ a 15-minute trip _____ 30-minute trip _____ a one-hour trip. Do you need access by public transportation? _____

◆ How long should it take to get an appointment for routine care if you have a medical condition that is not urgent, such as back pain? What do you think is reasonable? _____ 1–2 days _____ 3–5 days _____ 6–10 days

◆ How long should it take to get an appointment for a routine checkup or physical exam? _____ 1 week _____ 2–3 weeks_____ 4–6 weeks _____ 7–10 weeks

◆ How long should it take to get care when you are very sick, but it is not a medical emergency? _____ 1–4 hours _____ 5–8 hours _____ within 24 hours _____ within 2 days

◆ How long should it take to get your health questions answered by telephone? What do you think is reasonable? _____ within an hour _____ within a half day _____ the same day

◆ Would you like to be able to see different kinds of doctors and have lab and x-ray work done in one location? _____ What medical services that you frequently use would you want under one roof? _____

_____

◆ Are you interested in receiving preventive and routine medical care (for yourself or a child) from a nurse practitioner, physician's assistant, or other nonphysician medical professional if it means you can get an appointment sooner? _____

## Access to Care

One important indicator of quality in most people's minds is access; how easily and how quickly they can get the care they need. There are several kinds of access that are especially important to most consumers: how quickly they can get appointments and/or treatment when they are really sick; how quickly they can get convenient appointments for routine, nonurgent visits; how easily they can get through on the phone, especially when they have urgent medical concerns; and how long they will have to wait in their doctors' waiting rooms for scheduled appointments.

Many HMOs measure member satisfaction with access, or they may measure actual access times: how long it takes to get an urgent or routine appointment; how long a patient waits in the waiting room. This kind of information is most useful if you can compare one HMO's performance with another's. Your employer is likely to be the most reliable source, but the HMOs you are considering should also be willing and able to answer your questions about access. Let's take them one at a time.

### How Quickly Can You Get Urgent Treatment?

The rule here is very simple. You should be able to get care in a day or less if you have an urgent medical need. (This assumes that in the case of a medical emergency you will get immediate help.) Your HMO or HMO doctor should be able to offer same-day care to people who need it, either by keeping some appointment time open every day or through a special urgent care department. If your schedule for work, home, or child care limits the times of day you can conveniently come in for appointments, make sure you know your HMO doctor's office schedule. Is it open early in the morning, in the evening, and on weekends? Can you call at any time, twenty-four hours a day, and get the medical advice or the care you need?

### How Quickly Can You Get Routine Care?

Whether you belong to an HMO or not, you may feel that you should be able to get an appointment for a routine exam or nonurgent procedure within a few weeks or even days. Yet it is quite common for patients to face a four- to eight-week wait for some kinds of routine appointments. This is an area where communication is key: What are your expectations? What are the HMO's standards for routine appointments? Are there some doctors who have more flexibility in their schedules? Will you and your HMO doctor share the same idea of what is urgent and what is routine? Will your doctor's schedule be flexible enough for you to get an appointment on a date and at a time convenient to you?

### How Quickly Can You Get Through on the Phone?

If you call because you have an emergency, you should be able to get through to your doctor or HMO immediately.

Beyond that, it is likely to be a matter of personal tolerance. Many common medical problems can be handled over the phone, so you should be able to speak with a medical professional without having your patience tested by being on hold. In fact, access by phone should be something your doctor or HMO encourages. Some doctors schedule "call-in" time to guarantee their patients direct access for routine matters. Time on hold is a common problem for all service businesses these days, so automated systems are often used to direct calls or allow you to leave messages. What you probably want is a quick response from a real human being. Your HMO should be able to offer you that option in a timely manner—immediately, if you have a medical emergency.

### How Long Will You Wait in the Waiting Room?

The real question here is, How much can you stand? Most doctors, HMO or non-HMO, schedule more patients than they can possibly see on time and in time, because they can't predict which patients will not show up or exactly how long each patient will take. Ideally, you won't wait more than a half hour past your appointment time; you'll be told if and why you have to wait for more than fifteen minutes; you won't be put in a "holding room" (especially wearing a paper gown) in order to create the impression that you are no longer waiting; and you'll be given something to read besides ancient *Popular Mechanics*, *National Geographic*, or pharmaceutical magazines.

### Does the HMO Have Convenient Locations?

Convenience is largely a matter of personal preference. You may be willing to drive twenty or thirty minutes or more to an HMO clinic that meets your needs and has many services located under one roof. Or you may have to take your young children to a pediatrician frequently, so you prefer an HMO that has one near your home. You may require access by public transportation. Whatever your needs, you should be able to find out easily which HMOs can best meet them.

## OTHER THINGS TO CONSIDER

Once you have a pretty good idea how the HMO or HMOs available to you stack up in terms of cost, coverage, preventive care, physician choice, quality, and access, there are a few other important questions you should ask before you join.

### *Does the HMO Use Nonphysician Primary Care Clinicians?*

Many HMOs use primary care clinicians who are not doctors to take care of the more common, uncomplicated health needs of their members. Nurse practitioners (NPs) are registered nurses who have advanced degrees in an area of health care, such as pediatric or adult medicine, obstetrics/gynecology, or mental health care. They perform a wide range of primary care and preventive care functions and are highly skilled in counseling and health education. Physician's assistants (PAs) are graduates of a training and certification program that has been approved by the American Medical Association. They often evaluate, diagnose, and treat injuries, and assist with routine surgical procedures, all under the license and supervision of a doctor. In addition to PAs and NPs, HMO members may encounter a host of other clinical staff, including other nurses, physical and occupational therapists, speech and hearing therapists, and in some HMOs, certified nurse midwives, who provide care during pregnancies, labor, and birth, along with family planning and some types of gynecological care.

As an HMO member, you should always have a personal primary care doctor, but you may find that a nonphysician primary care clinician can meet most of your routine needs just as well, and may be available to you sooner than your doctor, either in person or over the phone. For instance, many people find that nurse practitioners are better able to meet their needs for counseling, advice, and health education—for the personal side of medical care—while their doctors can focus on the more technical aspects of care. Ideally, doctors and other clinicians should work in teams, and all members of the team should be trained in both the personal and technical aspects of medicine. The key is for all clinicians to know their limits—to know when they need to consult with someone with a more advanced or specialized level of knowledge to care for a patient. Before you join an HMO, you will want to understand whether, and under what circumstances, you are likely to see a nurse practitioner or physician's assistant rather than a doctor.

## Is the HMO Financially Stable?

When you join an HMO, you certainly want it to be there for you six months, a year, and two years from now. You don't want any surprises like benefit cuts or high premium increases. You don't want your doctor to have a negative attitude toward your HMO because he or she feels the HMO is failing to pay what it promised for medical services. In other words, you want your HMO to be financially stable.

Usually employers and government regulatory agencies keep close track of the financial condition of HMOs and can tell you if there are any problems that should concern you. Most states have financial safeguards in place so that if an HMO or other health plan faces bankruptcy the plan's members are protected for their care and coverage. But no one wants the uncertainty that comes with serious financial problems.

## *Is It a For-Profit or Not-for-Profit HMO?*

Is a for-profit HMO more likely to have a financial conflict of interest than a not-for-profit HMO; will the plan and its doctors withhold necessary care in order to increase their income and profits? This is a tough issue, and one for which you aren't likely to find an easy answer. While most of the early HMOs were not-for-profit organizations, many of the newer ones found it easier to raise start-up money by taking the for-profit route. And some not-for-profit HMOs are converting to for-profit status in order to attract new investment money.

Even not-for-profit HMOs have to maintain a "surplus," which is a profit by another name; the difference is that they aren't accountable to shareholders like for-profit HMOs. Instead, they set a portion of their surplus aside for future needs, or they use it to hold down their premiums. But since all HMOs are under intense pressure to keep costs down, not-for-profit status is no guarantee of better care. What's most important for you to keep in mind is that there are many ways for you to judge the quality of an HMO, and you have many allies, including employers and government regulators (and possibly your current doctor), to whom you can turn for information on HMO quality.

## *Does the HMO Offer Preenrollment Orientation Sessions?*

Some HMOs will hold orientations prior to enrollment. This means you will be able to visit their clinics or health centers, talk with doctors or other health professionals and member service representatives, and have your questions answered directly. While you may not think you have the time to attend such an orientation, it is a very good investment, given the financial and personal costs involved in making the wrong choice. It is an excellent way to get a feel for the HMO, and to gather more information on whether this HMO will meet your needs. Other useful alternatives are orientation videotapes or "welcome-call" orientations over the phone. Ask the HMO's member service department if preenrollment orientation is available.

## Can the HMO Meet Your Language and Diversity Needs?

Effective communication is at the heart of good health care. So much of what patients need has nothing to do with the technical aspects of medicine and everything to do with the human dimension. It is therefore very important that you feel you can communicate well with your health plan and with your doctor. If language is a potential barrier for you or any member of your family, if you or a dependent is physically or mentally challenged, or if ethnic, racial, or gender diversity is important to you, ask in advance whether and how the HMO will be able to meet your needs for access and communication.

## What Is the HMO's Word-of-Mouth Reputation?

One very useful piece of information in choosing an HMO is its reputation. In fact, most people say they would rather rely on the advice of their friends and neighbors in choosing a health plan than on what the HMO has to say about itself. So why is "word-of-mouth" at the end of this chapter instead of the beginning? Because, while friends and neighbors who belong to an HMO can help you with your decision, they should just be one source of information. The goal of this book is to make sure the HMO you choose meets your needs, and that you get the most out of your HMO membership. By this point in your reading and research, you should have a pretty good understanding of what your needs are, and what different HMOs offer. Your friends and neighbors probably have very different personal and medical needs, but they can be a very good "reality check" before you commit yourself to one plan or another.

You have to make sure you ask them the right questions, questions that cover your key issues and concerns. And, of course, the more people you ask, the more likely you are to get a well-rounded picture of how a particular HMO performs. You might ask: What are the five things you like best about HMO X? What are the five things you find most frustrating? Then ask yourself how these answers fit with what you were thinking. Do they raise any red flags that might make you want to reconsider or get more information before you make your decision?

# 3

## Becoming an HMO Member: Signing Up and Getting Started

Once you have asked all the right questions, and talked to all the right people, and made your decision about which HMO to join, it's time to apply for membership. What should you expect? First of all, you will need to fill out an application form, which you can get from your employer, government sponsor, or the HMO you have chosen. It's very important for you to fill it out completely and accurately. You don't want your HMO to lose track of you because you forgot to include some information. (Make sure you notify your HMO any time your address or phone number changes after you join.)

In most cases, when you apply through your employer, Medicare, or Medicaid, you will be automatically accepted for membership. Your "effective date" is the day when you will officially become a member; it can occur from several weeks to several months after you hand in your application. You will want to know exactly when the switch from your old coverage to your new plan takes place, especially if you are currently under medical care.

*Are You Asked to Choose a Doctor or a Health Care Site?*

An especially important part of the application process is choosing a doctor or a location (health center, clinic, medical group practice) where you will receive your primary care. Most IPAs will want you to choose your primary care doctor at the time you apply. Group or staff model plans may want you to choose a health care location; you will be asked to select a specific primary care doctor after you are enrolled. Filling out this information on your application will help get you connected to your HMO's health care network sooner. And remember, making a choice on your application doesn't mean you can't switch doctors or health care locations later on. (For more on choosing a doctor, turn to Chapter 4.)

*Are You Asked for Your Medical History?*

If you are enrolling directly, through a nongroup plan, you may have to fill out a more complicated application that includes a questionnaire on your past and current health status. You may even be asked to undergo a physical exam and submit a report from a doctor. All this is part of a health screening process for people who apply for the first time (they have not already been members through an employer group and converted from group to nongroup coverage). With health screening, the HMO can refuse membership or limit coverage for someone who has a history of poor health or who is at high risk for illness in the future. Some states prohibit health screening and limitations on coverage based on preexisting medical conditions.

## UNDERSTANDING WHO IS COVERED

Whether you are going to be covered through your employer, your spouse's employer, or directly, it is important to understand in advance who will be included in your HMO contract, and under what circumstances. Most HMOs use several terms to describe people covered under their contracts. The person who signs the application, who accepts the terms of the contract, and in whose name premiums are paid is the "subscriber." The subscriber and others who are covered by the HMO's contract are referred to as "members" or "enrollees."

HMOs usually offer two types of memberships: an individual membership that covers only a subscriber, and a family membership that covers the subscriber and one or more other family members. Some offer three options: an individual membership that covers only a subscriber, a two-person membership that covers the subscriber and one eligible family member, and a family membership that covers the subscriber and two or more other eligible family members.

You will find details in your contract about who is covered besides the subscriber. In general, coverage will include:

►The subscriber's spouse: The subscriber's husband or wife is covered if they have a family membership, or a two-person membership when it is available. If you get married while you are a member, your new spouse will become a member if you switch from an individual to a family (or two-person) membership. In the event of separation or divorce, the subscriber's separated or divorced spouse may continue to be covered until he or she remarries or drops coverage voluntarily, unless the separation or divorce judgment states otherwise, or coverage may end when the divorce takes effect. (State laws vary on the issue of coverage for separated or divorced spouses, so check your contract if this is a concern for you.)

►A limited number of employers and HMOs offer coverage for "domestic partners" or "spousal equivalents." This means two people who are in a long-term relationship without being legally married, and it may apply to homosexual couples only, or to both homosexual and heterosexual couples.

►Unmarried children: If you have a family membership (or one child and no spouse under a two-person membership), your dependent children under the age of nineteen are covered. It is important to enroll dependent children when you first join, otherwise you may not be able to do so until the next annual enrollment period. Newborn or newly adopted children can be added at the time of birth or adoption. You may also be able to get family coverage for children awaiting adoption, children for whom you are the legal guardian, and dependent stepchildren. When your children turn nineteen, they will no longer be covered under your contract, unless they are student dependents or disabled dependents. (This cutoff age may vary.)

►Student dependents: Unmarried student dependents who are enrolled full time in an accredited academic institution can usually have their coverage continued after their nineteenth birthdays. It is important to note that there will be a cutoff age for student dependent coverage, typically twenty-three or twenty-five years old, and your child's full-time student status will have to be verified each year. If your child graduates, drops out, switches to part-time studies, or reaches the cutoff age, coverage under your contract will end. Most HMOs will then offer your child the chance to convert to nongroup coverage. (Student coverage may be unavailable if you are a nongroup member of an HMO; if you have group coverage, the cutoff age will probably be decided by your employer.)

►Disabled dependents: Unmarried dependent children who are unable to support themselves because of mental or physical disability can be covered under the subscriber's family contract regardless of age. State laws vary on coverage for disabled dependents, so check your contract carefully.

## NEW MEMBER INFORMATION FROM YOUR HMO

Between the time you apply for membership and the effective date of your enrollment, you should receive some important information from your HMO. While everyone's natural tendency is to ignore this information or put it aside with the best intentions of getting to it later, you should take the time to understand what your HMO has sent you and why, and to read as much of the material as you can, or view your orientation video if you get one. (Many HMOs translate their orientation materials into languages other than English, so if you prefer another language, ask your HMO's member service department for help.) Take notes on anything you think is important for you and other members of your family to remember. If you still have questions, write them down. Don't throw anything away! You should receive from your new HMO:

▶A membership ID card or some other way for you to identify yourself as a member. You may or may not be asked to show your membership card whenever you see your HMO doctor, but you should always carry it with you in case you have an emergency or need care when you are traveling. It not only proves that you have insurance coverage, but will probably have information on it that is needed by any non-HMO doctors or hospitals that might have to care for you. Take a careful look at what is on your HMO membership card. Typically it will include your name and membership number; the name and phone number of your HMO doctor or HMO health center or clinic (or someplace to write it in);

information on benefits, such as your typical office visit fee, whether you have prescription drug coverage, and whether you are covered outside the HMO network; and information on what to do and who to call in an emergency. If you understand what is on your membership card and use that information appropriately, you will have gone a long way toward establishing a successful relationship with your HMO.

►Information on how to choose your primary care doctor. If you have not been asked to choose a doctor on your application form, you will receive a list of doctors from which to choose after you enroll, and information on how to choose a doctor and switch doctors if you want to later on.

►Information on where you will get your care and how. You should receive a complete guide on how to use your HMO, covering subjects ranging from how to schedule a routine appointment, to what will happen if you need to be hospitalized, to what to do in an emergency or when you need care when you are traveling. It should tell you what you need to do, and what your HMO will do for you, to make sure you get the care and coverage you need, whenever and wherever you need it.

►Information on what is covered and what, if any, copayments you'll have to pay when you get care. Your membership is based on a legal contract between you and your HMO or your HMO and your employer. That contract has probably been reviewed and approved by a state regulatory agency. It is the most complete description of your rights and responsibilities as a member. Since you will probably have to pay for any medical care that is not covered by your HMO, this contract is at the heart of a successful membership. Your member contract should be sent to you in its entirety or in detailed summary form, with information on how you can obtain a complete version of your contract. Since most HMOs offer many variations of their covered benefits, you may have amendments or riders attached to your contract that change your HMO's basic benefits in important ways. For instance, you may have riders that provide you with prescription drug coverage or dental care; require higher (or lower) visit fees or emergency room copayments than the "basic" benefit plan; or put limits on (or extend) the number of days certain types of treatment are covered. In other words, it is very important for you to read your contract or at least know where it is so you can look up benefits information in the future. It's a legal document, so you may find parts of it confusing, but most states require, and most HMOs want to offer, a contract that is in language that almost anyone can understand. If there is anything in your contract that is unclear to you, call your HMO's member service department or speak to your employer's health benefits administrator.

▶Information on your HMO's enrollment area or service area. The enrollment area is the geographical region in which members have to live to be eligible for coverage. Some plans have a different "service area," which includes additional communities surrounding the enrollment area. Sometimes the terms are interchangeable. This information should be found in your contract, which should include a map or a list of cities and towns. Most HMOs require you to play by different rules when you are inside your HMO's enrollment area or service area than when you are "out of area," so it is important to understand the boundaries. Since HMO enrollment and service areas can change as an HMO's physician network changes, you should always call your HMO before you travel, if you are not sure whether you will be outside their service area.

►Information on how to file claims for payment when you get care that is covered outside your HMO's network. This is especially important if you belong to a point-of-service plan that allows you to share the cost of non-network care.

►Information on how to get questions answered, file complaints, or appeal decisions on care or coverage. If you are in the dark about any aspect of your membership, you should be able to call someone for information. If you disagree with a decision by your HMO or HMO medical provider, you have the right to complain or file an appeal of that decision. In many cases, member appeals are decided in favor of the member, especially when the HMO has not done a good job of communicating what is expected or required of members. See Chapter 8, "Problems and Complaints," for more details.

►Information on advance directives such as living wills, health care proxies, or durable power of attorney. HMOs are required to inform their members about how they can plan for difficult health care decisions that might have to be made about them if they are seriously ill and unable to speak for themselves. The choices available to people vary according to different state laws, but in general people can and should discuss and plan with their families, doctors, and/or attorneys what kind of treatment they would want if they were terminally ill and unable to decide or communicate their decision at that time. You'll find more on this subject in Chapter 4.

►Information on special programs or features. Your HMO may offer some special programs that you will want to consider, such as health education and nutrition classes; discounts for fitness clubs and diet workshops; quit-smoking programs; discounted eyeglasses, carseats, bike helmets, and other health, fitness, and safety items; and orientations for new members. Other special features may include transportation services, translation services, special call-in times for your doctor, and twenty-four-hour hotlines.

All of this information should be kept in a single folder or envelope in a convenient and easily remembered place. You should keep your membership card and any children's cards in your wallet and post the HMO's emergency and member service numbers near your phone. Keep it all as long as you are a member or unless your HMO sends new information— a new membership card or new or amended contract, for instance—that supersedes the old information.

## IF YOU NEED CARE RIGHT AWAY

It's possible, of course, that you will get sick or injured even before your HMO has sent you its new member orientation materials or before you have chosen your primary care doctor. If you get sick and feel you need care right away, call your HMO doctor's office for advice or an appointment. If you have not yet chosen a primary care doctor, you have several choices:

▶If you have received a membership card but have not chosen a primary care doctor, look for the HMO phone number on the card and call before you get care. Your HMO will probably direct you to its urgent care department or help you choose a doctor, with whom you can then schedule an appointment. Some HMOs have special emergency phone numbers for you to call.

▶If you have not received any information from your HMO, but you know, or believe, that you are enrolled as a member, call your HMO's main phone number and ask for the member service department. It should be able to direct you to the care you need.

▶In either case, make sure you call first. If you get care
without calling for authorization from your HMO, except in
the case of an extreme emergency, you will probably have
to pay for it yourself.

## What If You Are Pregnant or Being Treated for a
## Serious Illness?

If you are pregnant or under treatment for a serious illness when you join an HMO for the first time or switch
HMOs, you are likely to feel anxious about both your care
and your coverage. Many HMOs have "clinical transition"
programs to help patients get connected to the HMO's network of specialists and hospitals without any break in their
care. Call your new HMO well in advance of your membership's effective date to find out how your case will be handled. Make sure you ask your current doctor or doctors to
help you with a smooth transition of your care to your
HMO.

If you are hospitalized on the effective date of your new
HMO coverage, your old insurer may be financially responsible for your hospital care for some period of time after the
effective date. That is a matter to be worked out by your old
insurer and your HMO; you should not have to worry about
any gaps in your care or your coverage unless there is a difference in benefits between your old and new plans. Here
too, check with your HMO's member service department
well in advance of the effective date of your HMO membership to confirm that there will be a smooth transition to
your new coverage. You'll find much more on dealing with
maternity and various illnesses in Chapter 7.

Find out if your HMO has a program to help patients
with medical problems make a smooth clinical transition
into the HMO. There may be "advice nurses" or other clinicians who can help you get the care or medications you need

as soon as you join, and can help you choose a primary care doctor. Call the member service department of your HMO (even before your membership takes effect, if possible), and ask if there is a clinical transition program or staff member who can help you with your specific medical needs.

Have your medical records transferred to your HMO. Submit a written request to your previous doctor or doctors and ask that a copy of your records be sent to you or your HMO doctor. If you have been hospitalized, your hospital records will probably be separate. Ask the hospital to send a copy of your discharge summary to you or your HMO. (If you have an especially complicated medical history, or if you have been cared for by many different doctors in many different places, your records may be scattered, complex, and difficult to read. If this is the case, ask your most recent physician to supply a summary of your care to date: your medical history, your current status, your treatment plan, important cautions and precautions, and any other important information.)

Schedule an appointment to meet with your primary care doctor as soon as convenient to review your health history and your current health status, and to discuss your needs, concerns, and preferences.

## What If You Need a Prescription Filled?

As soon as you have chosen a primary care doctor, you should call to discuss any ongoing medication needs you have. If you have not chosen a doctor or have not been contacted by your HMO, but you need a prescription, call your HMO's member service department to find out what you should do. (For more on prescription drug coverage, turn to Chapter 5.)

# 4

## Your HMO Doctor: Building a Partnership for Your Health

Not too long ago, most Americans were cared for by family doctors who could handle almost any medical condition from childbirth to the end of life. As medicine has become more advanced and technical, doctors have become more specialized, and there are now dozens of subspecialties covering all diseases and all parts of our bodies. The old-fashioned doctor who could do it all has become a rarity, but patients can still get personal, family-oriented care for most of their health needs. Today it's called primary care.

HMOs try to provide the most appropriate health care in the most appropriate setting. This is what allows them to offer a wide range of benefits at a reasonable price. In many cases, the most appropriate setting is in primary care, which is almost always less expensive than specialty or hospital care. Specialty care is important to our good health, but if it is overused, it can add unnecessary expense and make our medical care more fragmented and uncoordinated than it should be. So your HMO will want you to choose a primary care doctor who will take care of you. (Many HMOs use the term "primary care physician," or PCP.) The primary care doctors used by most HMOs include:

**Internists:** Physicians trained in the specialty of internal medicine, who care for adults.

**Pediatricians:** Physicians trained in the specialty of pediatric medicine, who care for children, generally up to age sixteen or eighteen.

**Family practitioners:** Physicians trained in the specialty of family practice, who care for patients of all ages and who can treat illnesses in areas ranging from pediatrics to geriatrics, from gynecology to cardiology.

Some HMOs allow "self-referral" to other selected specialties, like mental health, allergies, or dermatology, but that does not mean these specialties are considered primary care; members should still choose a primary care doctor. Also, gynecologists are considered primary care physicians in some HMO networks, which means women can make appointments directly, without a referral.

Primary care doctors often work in teams with other nonphysician primary care providers, like nurses and physician's assistants. You may be cared for by one of these health care professionals for more routine problems, such as conducting a physical exam, putting on a cast, stitching a cut, removing a mole, or instructing you how to manage an uncomplicated illness for yourself or a child. They also may handle arrangements before and after a hospitalization or help with issues like family planning, nutrition, and management of chronic illnesses, such as diabetes, and they can provide care and advice in many other situations. In some states they may even be authorized to write certain prescriptions.

# THE MANY ROLES OF
# YOUR PRIMARY CARE DOCTOR

Whether you need immediate treatment for an injury or illness (if it is not life threatening), a routine checkup, a Pap test or mammogram, care for chronic back pain, or a prescription for your allergies, you're likely to get most of your care from your HMO primary care doctor. Your primary care doctor has several roles:

▶Caregiver: The most important role for your primary care doctor is to be your personal doctor and to provide the medical care you need when you are sick or injured. Whether it is by giving advice over the telephone, by seeing you in the doctor's office, or by placing you in the care of another member of the clinical team, your primary care doctor should be able to handle most of your medical needs. If you are joining an HMO for the first time, you may have been seeing a specialist whom you considered to be your personal doctor—someone who practices at an excellent hospital, who knows "all the best people" in the medical community, who was all you really needed. If you take the time to choose carefully and work to establish a good relationship, you should be able to find an HMO primary care physician who can meet the same high standards.

▶Counselor and consultant: A successful doctor-patient relationship is often more dependent on good communication than on medical technology. Your HMO primary care doctor should be someone who can make you feel that your needs for information, as well as medical care, are being met. It is not just a case of good "bedside manner"; your doctor should be able to explain what he or she is, or is not, doing in a way that says, "We share an interest in your good health and well-being." Your primary care doctor must also act as a consultant and coordinator, pulling together the various parts of the medical community that are available to you when you need them, making sure that neither you nor information about your medical treatment falls through the cracks.

►Gatekeeper: Some HMOs describe their primary care doctors as "gatekeepers." This is another way of saying that your primary care doctor controls your access to specialists, to hospitals or other medical resources, and to anyone outside the HMO network. Generally this means that you will have to receive a "referral" or authorization from your HMO doctor, in writing or over the phone, in order for you to receive the care and/or be covered. Your personal HMO doctor should be able to meet most of your medical needs, but if she can't, she should "open the gate" to other resources and direct you to the care you need. Your primary care doctor should take an active role, and assume responsibility for coordinating all of your care, even if she does not provide it directly. The last thing you want is for your doctor or HMO to be a barrier, a "guardian of the gate," between you and medical care. On the other hand, you should not simply view your primary care doctor as someone who writes referrals so you can see the specialist of your choice. You and your doctor need to develop a relationship based on mutual trust and respect.

►Advocate: Ideally, you want a doctor who is your partner in good health, someone who makes decisions in partnership with you based on what is necessary and appropriate for you, and who communicates those decisions in a way that suits you. And, of course, someone who has the medical skills to provide or arrange for the best-quality care.

You also want a doctor who is not at odds with your HMO, someone who understands and accepts how the HMO works, and who is trusted and valued by the HMO for his or her medical judgment and quality as well as for the ability to make decisions that are cost effective.

What happens, then, if your doctor's medical judgment comes into conflict with what the HMO covers in your benefits contract? What if your doctor thinks you should have a type or amount of treatment that is not covered? This is a dilemma your doctor should be willing and able to negotiate without putting you in the middle. The more he or she feels like a partner with the HMO, rather than like someone whose medical decisions are "reviewed" or "policed" by the HMO based on cost alone, the more likely it is that this kind of conflict can be avoided.

## CHOOSING YOUR PRIMARY CARE DOCTOR

In choosing a doctor, you are looking for a person with a combination of medical expertise and personal qualities that will work for you. Determining who offers the right combination will probably entail some work, but it will be worth the effort.

Even if you don't have any immediate medical needs at the time you join an HMO, you should choose a primary care doctor as soon as possible. If you don't, you may find yourself facing needless delay or in a situation where a doctor is assigned to you if you need care. And remember, in most cases, the services of other providers are covered only when there has been a referral or authorization from your primary care doctor.

Depending on the type of HMO you join, you will choose your primary care doctor either before or after you apply. If you have a doctor you like and trust who is on the HMO's list of participating primary care doctors, you may simply choose to stick with him or her. Or you may want to, or have to, choose a new doctor. About two of every five new HMO members change doctors when they join.

Every HMO will provide new members with a list of its primary care doctors from whom to choose. This list is a good starting point, but may not provide as much information as you might want to make a truly informed and confident choice. Many HMOs have staff whose job it is to help you make your decision. And you may want to do a little research on your own. Make sure you find out if any of the doctors on the list are not accepting new patients or if they have waiting lists. An HMO should tell you this in advance if at all possible, but, just in case, you should be prepared to make a second choice if your first-choice doctor is not available.

## Interviewing the Doctor

When you think about it, you are "hiring" your personal doctor to perform a very important, very personal, and very expensive service for you. So a thorough job interview should not seem unreasonable. Call the doctor's office and ask to schedule a brief meeting or some telephone time. If that's impossible, explain that you are in the process of choosing a primary care physician, and ask to speak with someone who can give you accurate and thorough answers. Use the "Health Needs Assessment" questionnaires you filled out in Chapter 2 to focus on the issues that are most important to you. A key to a good medical relationship is good communication, so a doctor who will not answer your questions before taking you on as a patient may not be able to meet your needs.

Here are some of the things you will want to know in order to find the best doctor for you and other family members.

## *What Are the HMO Doctor's Credentials?*

Some HMOs will furnish you with background information on all of their doctors; HMOs with a large network of participating physicians are much less likely to do so. If you don't get anything in writing from the HMO, call the HMO's member service department or the doctor's office for help.

▶Medical training: You may feel more comfortable with a doctor who has been trained at a well-known medical school or who has been trained locally. But remember, the United States certainly doesn't have a monopoly on good medical training, and foreign-trained doctors have to meet the same standards as anyone else who is licensed to practice in this country.

▶Experience: How long a doctor has been practicing may be important to you, but with medical technology and training changing so rapidly, a young doctor may be just as competent as a more experienced one.

▶Board certification: A doctor who is board certified has pursued advanced training in his or her specialty, and has passed a qualifying examination; a doctor who is board eligible has received the training but has not taken or passed the exam. This is not the same as being licensed; a doctor without a license cannot legally practice medicine. At a minimum, your doctor should be board eligible.

▶Malpractice or disciplinary actions: Mistakes are made in medicine, just as in any other profession. But in medicine, a person's health, well-being, or ability to function is usually at stake—sometimes a person's life. Doctors who lose malpractice cases, or who reach out-of-court settlements, are not necessarily bad doctors. However, a pattern of multiple cases brought could mean trouble. Check with your state's board of medical registration for records of disciplinary actions against physicians for physical or sexual abuse of patients or problems with drugs, alcohol, or fraud.

►Sex and race: First and foremost for some people is whether their doctor is a man or woman. That should be pretty easy to determine, although some names are ambiguous. If race is important, you will probably have to ask.

## Where Are the HMO's Doctors Located?

Ideally, your HMO will have doctors located near where you live or near where you or your spouse works. If you join an HMO that has doctors practicing in health centers, clinics, or medical group practices, you will probably be asked first to choose a location, then a doctor. You can choose a different location or doctor for each member of your family if that is most convenient for you. If a plan has a mix of doctors practicing in clinics or groups and those practicing in private offices, you will want to decide which is more convenient to you, having your primary care doctor very close by, or being able to have access to a number of different medical services under one roof.

## Will You Be Able to Get Care When You Need It?

A good doctor is not much use to you if you can't get access to care when you need it. You'll want to know about appointment scheduling, office hours, what happens when your doctor's office is closed, and how and where you will be taken care of for medical problems that are beyond the scope of your primary care doctor's practice. The only way to get information on these topics is to ask either the doctor, the doctor's office staff, or your HMO. Some of this information may be available in written form from your HMO or your employer, but is likely to be general rather than specific to each doctor. And, of course, asking will give you an idea about how responsive the doctor or doctor's staff will be in the future. Here are some questions to ask:

►How long will it take you to get an appointment if you are very sick (if your child is very sick)? For a same-day appointment, are you likely to be seen by another member of the doctor's clinical team? Does that matter to you? If so, ask what the policy is.

►How long will it take to get an appointment for a routine examination or for a medical condition that is not urgent? First of all, you want to understand in advance how your doctor will define "urgent." Otherwise you may be very dissatisfied when this situation does arise. There is no "right" answer to the question of how long it should take to schedule a routine appointment. It may be a week or two, or a month or two. What feels right to you, and how well your doctor's office responds to your sense of urgency, will be most important.

►What is the doctor's policy for canceled appointments? Most require notification twenty-four hours in advance if at all possible. Ask if the appointment waiting time will start all over again if you cannot keep your first appointment.

►What will happen if you have an urgent medical problem at a time when your doctor's office is not open? You will want to be assured that you will have quick access to medical advice around the clock, seven days a week. This is especially important since you are required to call before seeking medical care, except in a serious emergency. Some HMOs have twenty-four-hour emergency hotlines, special centralized referral services, or phone systems that can direct member calls to an emergency service when the doctor's office or clinic is closed. These "after-hours" services are usually staffed by nurses or other medical professionals who have been trained in urgent and emergency care. Many doctors have answering services and backup systems for covering their practices around the clock. Especially if you have young children or old or chronically sick family members, you will want to know exactly who will get back to you, and how quickly, if you call about a crisis in the middle of the night.

►What hospital will you be sent to? Except in extreme emergencies, all hospitalizations for HMO members have to be authorized in advance by their primary care physicians or by approved HMO specialists. Your HMO will provide you with a list of "affiliated hospitals" in their marketing or member literature. That list may be too general, however, to tell you where your primary care doctor or HMO specialist would hospitalize you or members of your family. Your HMO may have many hospital affiliations, and where you are hospitalized often depends on what you need. You should ask where you might be admitted for major or complex surgical procedures; for less serious problems like appendicitis or a broken hip; for childbirth; for surgery that does not require an overnight stay, such as hernia repair or cataract surgery; and for specialized hospitalization, such as for cancer treatment, rehabilitation, mental illness, or substance abuse.

►What specialist will you be referred to if you have a medical problem your primary care doctor cannot handle? HMOs may have "in-house" specialists or they may have preferred specialists in the community. They could also leave specialty referrals entirely up to the discretion of the physician. If you have a medical problem that requires the ongoing attention of a specialist, you will want specific information on whom your primary care doctor will refer you to, what role you'll have in that decision, and how the referral will be arranged. If you are referred to someone you don't know, you will want to ask many of the same questions about access and quality you would ask when choosing a primary care doctor. Finding out who are *thought* to be the leading specialists in your community may be easy; just ask around. Finding out who is really the best is much more difficult.

CASE EXAMPLE:
CHOOSING A NEW DOCTOR

*Lorraine was fifty-six years old when she joined an HMO for the first time. She was concerned that her former doctor didn't participate in the HMO, so that she had to choose a new primary care doctor. She was very interested in women's health issues and she had a strong preference for an older, female doctor like her former doctor. After checking her HMO's doctor list, Lorraine found that there were only two female doctors in the group practice that was closest to her home. One was a recent medical school graduate, and the other was so popular that she had stopped accepting new patients. What should Lorraine do?*

*Lorraine decided that it was well worth her time to do some more research. She realized that she had several options available to her. She could ask her HMO if the older woman had a waiting list for patients that she could be put on if she chose another doctor in the meantime. She could ask if her HMO would allow her to choose a gynecologist as her primary care physician for women's health issues if she could find a female gynecologist who practiced nearby. The group practice she'd chosen had several female nurse practitioners, one of whom could be her primary care provider for routine problems and for counseling about women's health issues, so that was an option. And she could even ask her former doctor if she would consider joining the HMO's network; that way, Lorraine could continue to see her.*

*Lorraine decided her first step should be to ask some friends and coworkers if any of them were patients of the younger woman doctor. When she found out that several were, and that they liked her, she called the doctor's office and scheduled a brief phone interview. She asked about some issues that were very important to her, and, much to her delight, she felt immediately comfortable with the doctor's manner and her knowledge. Knowing that she could switch later if she wanted to, Lorraine chose the younger woman as her primary care doctor. She also found out that her HMO had some special programs for women's health, including prevention, screening, and health education, and she worked with her primary care doctor to make sure she could participate in the ones that interested her.*

## HOW TO TALK WITH YOUR DOCTOR

Playing by the rules of your HMO won't guarantee that you will feel totally comfortable with the health care you receive. That takes personal involvement in decisions about your care and good communication with your caregivers, starting with your personal doctor. It's not that hard, if you prepare yourself. That's what this section is all about.

Even when you've done all you can to choose the right doctor and picked someone you feel really good about, funny things can happen when you step into your doctor's office. Even the calmest person can feel a twinge of anxiety. Questions you definitely meant to ask suddenly fade from memory. You're left tongue-tied, and the best comment you can offer is "Yes, doctor, I understand."

It's a common reaction and probably just as frustrating to your doctor as it is to you. Effective communication is a responsibility shared by you and your doctor. You need to make sure you are clear about why you scheduled an appointment and what you expect from your doctor. You need to do more than present a problem; you need to ask for help. Your doctor should make sure you are satisfied and that you understand what is being discussed and what you have to do after the appointment.

Very often, the reason you don't talk with your doctor as well as you could is that you simply aren't sure what to ask. But there are some basic questions you can ask when you need routine care, and when you are sick or need surgery. Familiarizing yourself with these questions now may prepare you for those unsettling moments when you know you want more information, or a clearer explanation, from your primary care clinician or a specialist.

And remember, these questions apply not only to you but to any member of your family, or to anyone who relies on you to help interpret and follow a doctor's advice.

## Getting Comfortable with Your Doctor

You are waiting in the exam room, sitting on the crisp white sheet of paper covering the exam table, with half your clothes off and your legs dangling over the side. You are cold, but you are sweating. You are anxious. Will your doctor find nothing wrong with you and think you wasted her time? Or will your problem be even more serious than you thought? In walks your doctor, who you know is very busy and who you find a little intimidating. It's a hard way to begin a dialogue.

One way to break the ice is with small talk. Even a simple "How are you today?" will give your doctor a chance to interact with you in a more personal way. If you are still uncomfortable or nervous, don't be afraid to say so. Just getting it off your chest will help. Once you and your doctor relax, you can quickly move to the reason for your visit.

As you start talking about your medical problem, make

sure you try to address all of your concerns up front, with as much detail as possible. For example, don't just say, "My stomach hurts a lot." Try to track your discomfort more carefully and see if you can be more helpful: "For the past three weeks, I've been getting a sharp pain on my right side about an hour after I eat."

If you think you know what is wrong with you, or have some particular fear in your mind, say so: "My mother had a lot of trouble with gallstones and I'm concerned that my pain might be gallstones." Or, in a different case: "I've had terrible headaches for the past two weeks and I'm afraid I might have a brain tumor because I've never had headaches before." That will give your doctor a chance to immediately address, and probably rule out, your greatest fears. It will help her know what questions to ask you in her step-by-step diagnosis.

## What You Should Bring to a Doctor's Appointment

It helps if you come to your appointment with a written list of your symptoms and your questions. If you have been taking medications or undergoing treatment, write those details down before your appointment. You may want to bring your medications with you.

On your first visit, you should also plan to talk to your doctor or other clinician about your family history, stressful factors in your life, illnesses you've had in the past, and your personal health-related habits. This information is very important in getting your care off to a good start, and it will all be confidential, so you should be as open and complete as possible.

## Questions for a Routine Visit

Even with a routine or preventive-care visit such as a checkup, you should be ready to ask your doctor some important questions. If you're like most of us, though, the real problem isn't how to ask but what to ask. In the course of your visit, you will want to know:

◆ What will your doctor check for at each routine visit?
◆ What tests will be performed and why? These can include blood pressure, a urine test, one for blood in your stool, and routine blood tests, particularly for cholesterol.
◆ How often does your doctor plan to repeat any tests and why?
◆ When and how will your test results be reported to you, and what can you expect if the test detects a possible problem?
◆ Will you get any immediate test results, plus an explanation of those results?
◆ How does your health compare on this visit to previous visits (if this is not your first visit)? If your doctor mentions any changes, be sure to ask why these may have occurred and if anything should be done about them.
◆ Is there any medical information that your doctor feels you should have on hand at all times? It may also be important for you to discuss your normal blood pressure range and cholesterol count, as well as any chronic condition you may have. Knowing, for example, that you've had a "functional" heart murmur since childhood could save you unnecessary testing in the future.

In short, the right questions—and the right answers—should uncover a great deal about your health and the factors that affect it. Get in the habit of asking what you and your doctor can do, together, to protect your health, and how. Once you become an active participant in your own medical well-being, you can expect to better understand any care you may receive.

CASE EXAMPLE:
IS MY HMO REALLY COMMITTED TO PREVENTION?

*When Marie changed jobs, she joined an HMO, and she was pleased that she didn't have to change doctors. But she was soon confused. Under her old insurance plan, she had a general physical exam every year. As a matter of fact, her old company had encouraged high-level executives like herself to have annual physicals, and they paid the full cost for senior managers who had traditional health insurance. Recently, her doctor's office sent her a notice to come in for her annual physical. But her new HMO's prevention guidelines say that a woman of her age, thirty-eight, should have a general physical only every five years; what she needed every year were certain specific screening tests. She joined the HMO because she believes in prevention and in keeping health care costs down. What should Marie do?*

*Marie was caught in a conflict between what is considered by her HMO to be the best practice for people in general and what her doctor may think is right for her. The prevention guidelines used by many HMOs have been developed by physicians, using evidence gathered nationally regarding how appropriate and useful specific preventive practices are for large and diverse groups of people. Marie and her doctor need to agree on what is appropriate in her individual case, based on her medical risks and preferences.*

*There is no documented evidence that a complete head-to-toe physical examination is useful to preventive care. However, there are specific parts of a routine checkup that are of proven value in the early detection or prevention of disease. Another important purpose of a routine visit is that it gives the patient and doctor an opportunity to discuss health-related behaviors, such as diet, smoking, and exercise.*

*Marie decided to use her physical-exam appointment to talk with her doctor about her HMO's prevention guidelines, especially those that are important to women of her age, such as breast exams, mammography, Pap smears, and blood pressure measurement. She found out that her doctor considers her to be at high risk, and that's why he wanted to screen her more often than the HMO recommended. Her doctor told her he would take responsibility for making sure her HMO would cover her screenings. This was a good opportunity for Marie to get involved in some important decisions about her health care, and to plan with her doctor for her future preventive care.*

## Questions When You Are Sick

Diarrhea, common colds, bumps and bruises, yeast infections, poison ivy—these types of conditions are often easily treated by over-the-counter medications you can buy without a prescription, or by simply resting and waiting. So in many cases, you won't even need to call or see your HMO doctor. Of course, if you aren't sure what home remedy or over-the-counter drug is best, or if symptoms persist or get worse, you should call your doctor's office for advice. You may be asked to come in for an appointment, or your doctor may recommend a prescription medication. Here are some key issues to consider:

◆ If your doctor is very busy, is there a nurse or some other qualified medical professional who can take care of your routine medical problems or give you advice?

◆ Does your HMO offer or recommend books or courses on self-care for simple medical problems?

◆ Does your HMO have a special service for phone advice about routine problems?

◆ Does your doctor have a special call-in time for phone advice about simple medical problems?

If over-the-phone advice and over-the-counter remedies aren't enough, you'll need an appointment. Unfortunately, the hardest time to communicate is when you feel sick. You are probably uncomfortable and tired, and you may be frightened. But that's when the right questions can be the most important. Here are some tips for talking about a medical problem, either to your primary care doctor or a specialist.

Once you've stated your problem as clearly as you can, and given your doctor time to ask his or her own questions, perform an examination, and conduct any tests that might be necessary to reach a diagnosis, it's time for your questions.

◆ What does the diagnosis mean? What isn't working right—and why? Don't stop asking until you understand.

◆ What caused the problem? It's possible to prevent many diseases or conditions from happening again. Eating the wrong types of foods, smoking, maintaining a lifestyle that doesn't support your good health are just a few possibilities. If you don't ask about causes, you may never find a solution.

◆ What further tests should be done and what can you
   hope to learn from them?
◆ Does your doctor or HMO have any literature you can use
   to learn more about your illness and how to control it?

Just remember, when something's wrong, it's more important than ever that you keep the lines of communication
with your doctor open. Be sure you understand any diagnosis, any treatment, and any effects—good or bad—that those
treatments will have.

## Understanding What to Do Next

Once you have a clear idea of what's wrong, you'll want to
know what your doctor plans to recommend and how you
can help with your recovery. Sometimes the solution is obvious, but many times there are several options. Whatever the
case, you should ask what treatment your doctor thinks is
best and why.

◆ If your doctor is going to refer you to a specialist, who
   will you see; why was that doctor chosen; what should
   you expect from the referral visit; and what should you
   do to make sure it is covered by your health plan?
◆ If medication is prescribed, why do you need it and what
   is it supposed to do? Find out about possible side effects
   and adverse reactions and what you should do if you
   experience any of these. Make sure you know how to
   take your medication—with meals or on an empty stomach. Ask if it's safe to use your medication along with
   common over-the-counter medications, such as aspirin
   or antihistamines. And don't forget to mention any other
   prescription medication you're taking.

- Once you begin treatment, what signs will indicate that your treatment is—or isn't—working?
- How soon can you expect your treatment to bring relief, particularly if your problem is marked by pain, swelling, or any other sign you can monitor?
- When should you contact your doctor so he or she can monitor your progress?

When you really understand your treatment, the reasons for it, and how soon you can expect to feel better, you're better able to work with your doctor toward good health. If, at the end of an appointment, you haven't gotten what you need, either in terms of information or clear direction, *speak up*! You may want to schedule another appointment or speak to someone else on your doctor's clinical team, like a nurse who can spend more time with you, or with whom you might communicate more effectively.

## When You Need Surgery

If your personal doctor determines that surgery is necessary, he or she may refer you to a surgeon. Talking with a surgeon is often more intimidating than talking with your primary care physician, especially since the two of you may be meeting for the first time. All the more reason, though, to pull out your list of questions. You will want to know:

- Is surgery really necessary and what are the alternatives, if any?
- What risks are involved?
- What is the surgeon's experience in this procedure?
- What will happen if you don't have the surgery?

If you decide surgery is your best solution, you'll want to know:

◆ Will you have to be hospitalized or can the surgery be performed in an ambulatory surgery facility?

◆ How long will your recovery period be, what signs of recovery should you look for, and how long a stay can you expect in the hospital?

◆ What should you expect when you wake from surgery, how will you feel, where will you be, what equipment or tubes will be attached to you? Know as much as you can in advance so you won't be in a panic when you wake up.

◆ Are there any trouble signs you should look for after you leave the hospital, and what troubling signs are really a normal part of your healing process?

Once you get into the habit of asking questions about your health care, no matter how difficult or probing those questions may be, you establish yourself as a patient with whom doctors can discuss treatments and expect thoughtful and cooperative decisions.

If you prepare yourself to ask the right questions, it will be much easier to talk with your doctor or to anyone else your doctor recommends. At first, you may be surprised to discover just how much more information your doctor shares with you. It might seem a little overwhelming, but once you get used to being an involved and informed patient, you will realize how much more comfortable you are with your health care.

## GETTING A SECOND OPINION

As an HMO member, you have the right to get a second opinion if you are unsure about the diagnosis or the treatment recommended by your doctor. Even if you have established a relationship of trust and open communication with your doctor, asking for a second opinion may be uncomfortable for you. It is not easy to question your doctor's professional judgment.

Just keep two things in mind: First, medicine is not an exact science; there is not always a right or wrong answer. Second, you have the absolute right and responsibility to be involved in decisions affecting your health and well-being. So you must be sure that you understand why a particular type of treatment is being recommended and what the expected outcome will be. And if you are not satisfied with what you hear from your doctor, you should always ask for a second opinion. What you need to do to get a second opinion may vary somewhat from plan to plan. Ask your doctor, or, if you are not comfortable doing that, ask your HMO's member service department to help you.

In most cases, second opinions fall under the same rules as other HMO care and coverage. In other words, you will have to be referred by your HMO or HMO doctor for a second opinion, and you will have to get a second opinion from a doctor who is part of your HMO's network unless you have the right to go outside the network. Of course you may get a second opinion (or third opinion) from anyone you choose, without authorization or referral from your HMO, if you are willing to pay for it yourself. And if the outside opinion differs from that of your HMO doctor, you may be able to use the information to change or appeal your HMO's recommended course of treatment. What you should *not* do is proceed with treatment based on an outside second opinion and then expect your HMO to pay for it. Always use your HMO's member service and appeals process if you disagree with a care or coverage decision. Otherwise, you may be responsible for the full cost of your care. (See Chapter 8 for more information on how to handle appeals.)

If you belong to a point-of-service HMO, you can get a second opinion under your plan's non-network rules, and pay the extra amount required for it to be covered.

## Your Right to Refuse Treatment

There may also be times when, for personal or religious reasons, you don't want to follow the treatment recommendations of your HMO doctor. You have the right to accept or refuse a treatment or procedure before it has started and to have treatment stopped after it has begun. (Your exact rights may depend on the laws of your state.) If you decide to refuse treatment, your HMO will not be responsible for the medical consequences of your decision or for the cost of any alternative treatment you choose for yourself. You should also find out if your HMO will cover treatment for medical problems that occur because you refused to follow your HMO doctor's initial treatment recommendations.

Your doctor has the responsibility to explain clearly and thoroughly what all of your treatment options are, and what the expected consequences would be, before you decide what to do. Your decision should be well informed and it should be voluntary.

If your religious beliefs affect the type of medical care you are willing to accept, you should take the time to discuss this with your HMO's member service department before you join, and with your HMO doctor after you join.

# PREPARING FOR
# DIFFICULT HEALTH CARE DECISIONS

You also have the right to decide what treatment you want, or don't want, and who should make decisions about your treatment if you are unable to decide or speak for yourself because of a very serious illness or accident. If you want to be a full participant in medical decisions about your care, you will need to make your wishes known in advance.

Modern medicine is capable of keeping people alive even when they are terminally ill or hopelessly incapacitated with no chance of recovery. So it is possible that you will someday be a candidate for life-saving or life-sustaining treatments, such as cardiopulmonary resuscitation (CPR), mechanical breathing on a respirator, artificial feeding (nutrition and fluids given through a tube), kidney dialysis, or intensive hospital care. These are sometimes referred to as "extreme measures" if a patient's condition is thought to be terminal or irreversible.

Some people would want to keep these treatments to a minimum, or have them withheld altogether. They would prefer to avoid treatments or procedures that delay the inevitable, cause prolonged suffering or unnecessary expense, or rob them of their dignity. Other people would choose to have everything possible done to keep them alive, either because they would hold out the hope for recovery or because they believe life is sacrosanct and should be sustained at any cost. Whatever your point of view may be, you have a much better chance of getting what you want if you act in advance.

The most common ways to prepare for these difficult health care decisions are by using "advance directives" (written instructions about your wishes), including a living will, and by appointing a health care agent (sometimes called "health care proxy" or "durable power of attorney for health care"). Your ultimate rights in this area will be governed by the laws of your state. For instance, living wills and health care agents have more legal authority in some states than in others. In general, they work like this:

▶Living wills: A living will is a document that allows you to write down specific instructions about future medical treatment. Your instructions must be very clear and precisely stated in order for them to be useful if a medical crisis occurs. If you would like to prepare a living will, ask your HMO doctor or HMO if they have a standard form that you can use. You don't need a lawyer to prepare one.

You will need to sign your living will and have it witnessed by several people (not relatives, your doctor, or anyone who could benefit from your estate). Your doctor and members of your family should have copies of your living will; ask your HMO if anyone else should have copies. Since it is difficult to anticipate in advance every possible circumstance in which someone might have to make a difficult decision about taking extreme measures on your behalf, you may want to appoint a health care agent who understands how you generally feel about such issues.

►Health care agent, proxy, or durable power of attorney for health care: In many states you may formally appoint someone as your health care agent, which means they can make health care decisions for you in the event you cannot. (A few states allow family members to participate in these decisions without being formally appointed in advance.) You can appoint a health care agent by completing a legal form that names a substitute decision-maker. This is sometimes called a "health care proxy form" or "durable power of attorney for health care form." (But that doesn't necessarily mean an attorney has to be involved.) This form allows your health care agent to act for you only if your doctor determines—in writing—that you are unable to make or communicate your own health care decisions. Your health care agent would then have the legal authority to make decisions for you, including decisions about life-sustaining treatment (subject to state laws).

►Obviously it is important that whomever you choose to be your health care agent should be someone you trust and someone who understands how you feel about life-sustaining treatment. It cannot be your doctor, but it can be a member of your family or a friend. The form you fill out to designate a health care agent will specify what powers you want him or her to have, what specific limitations you might want to put on your agent's authority, and any other information you want to include about your point of view and values. You can include a living will as part of this document. You will have to sign the forms and have them notarized or witnessed, and make sure your doctor, members of your family, and your health care agent have copies.

Remember, you can revise or withdraw your living will or health care agent forms at any time if you change your mind about how you want these decisions made for you.

# 5

## Getting the Care and Coverage You Need: Emergency Care, Specialty Care, Out-of-Town Care, and More

When you join an HMO, especially when you join one for the first time, it is important to know how to get started—how to get the care and coverage you need from the first day of your membership. Even if you don't have any immediate medical needs, there are some things you should do to make sure you know how to "use the system." Many problems that HMO members have—problems that lead to confusion, miscommunication, and sometimes added expense—occur at the start of a new membership or when a member needs medical care for the first time. As you've already seen, there are important differences between the way HMOs work and what you might be used to if you have been covered by traditional insurance. Learning a few basic rules of HMO membership will get you off to a good start and help you get the most out of your HMO from day one. There are three areas that seem to cause HMO members the most headaches:

- ◆ Understanding what to do in a medical emergency.
- ◆ Getting specialty care with a referral from your primary care doctor.
- ◆ Knowing what to do if you need medical care when you are traveling away from home.

This chapter will equip you with guidelines you should follow and questions you should ask to get the most out of your HMO, for these and some other situations, including hospitalization and some potential problem areas, like cosmetic surgery and alternative therapies. These guidelines apply whether you have:

▶a standard HMO plan that restricts your coverage to those services that are provided or arranged by your HMO or HMO doctor (in-network services), or

▶a point-of-service HMO plan that gives you full coverage for services that are provided or arranged by your HMO (in-network services) and also allows you to arrange your own care, at a higher cost to you, with any provider outside the HMO's network. However, if you have a point-of-service HMO plan, the information in this chapter applies to your in-network care only. Advice on how to get the most from your non-network care can be found in the next chapter.

## GETTING CARE IN AN EMERGENCY

We all know what a medical emergency is: it's when you need immediate medical attention. We all know—or can imagine—what we'd feel in an emergency: fear, panic, pain, impatience. But when it comes to HMO care and coverage, there are two types of "medical emergencies," urgent and life-threatening, and understanding the difference between them is essential to determining how your care is handled and whether it will be paid for. Urgent care situations require you to call your HMO or HMO doctor in advance; in a life-threatening emergency you don't have to call before getting help.

## Urgent Care

Some medical problems require urgent attention or advice. A high fever that suddenly rises, a severely sprained ankle or a broken bone, a very sore throat or earache accompanied by high fever, uncontrolled vomiting, a cut that may need stitches—all are examples of situations that may be frightening or painful, but are usually not life-threatening. So any time, day or night, the first step is to call your doctor's office or your HMO's urgent care number. You will be told what to do and where to go for treatment. By following this simple procedure, you can be sure you are covered because your HMO doctor or HMO will have provided or authorized your care. You may have to pay a copayment if you are authorized to go to a hospital emergency room for treatment, but that copayment will probably be waived if you are admitted to the hospital. Here are some key issues to consider:

◆ Do you know what number to call if you need urgent care? Do you know what number to call when your doctor's office is closed?

◆ Do you know where you might be told to go for care when your doctor's office is closed? Do you know how to get there?

◆ If you are told to go to an emergency room, will you have to pay a copayment if you are not admitted to the hospital? How much?

◆ Does your HMO have an urgent care or drop-in service that allows you to go in without calling in advance?

◆ When you receive authorized urgent care from someone other than your HMO doctor, are you expected to notify your HMO? Should you expect your HMO doctor to take responsibility for your follow-up care?

## SERIOUS (LIFE-THREATENING) MEDICAL EMERGENCIES

If you have a very serious illness or injury that, if not treated right away, could result in death, permanent disability, disfigurement, or a severe long-term medical problem, you should get immediate medical assistance, without first calling your HMO doctor or HMO for authorization. Instead, you should call 911 or your local seven-digit medical-emergency phone number for emergency medical assistance, or else go or be taken to the nearest hospital emergency room. When you call for help, state that you have a medical emergency, what kind of emergency it is, who you are, and where you are located.

If you use an emergency room for care of a medical problem that is not a serious or life-threatening emergency, and you were not given authorization in advance by your HMO doctor or HMO, you may be responsible for paying all charges related to your emergency room care (and ambulance, if one was used).

Given the potential cost of using an emergency room when you shouldn't, it's important to understand how your HMO defines urgent versus life-threatening emergencies. Some typical examples HMOs use to define serious or life-threatening emergencies that don't require you to call before getting care include:

◆ Indications of a possible heart attack, such as chest pains and shortness of breath

- Indications of a possible stroke, such as loss of consciousness, vision, speech, or feeling
- Suspected poisoning or drug overdose
- Loss of consciousness due to a blow to the head
- Convulsions
- Inability to breathe
- Uncontrollable bleeding
- Crushing injuries
- Multiple or severe fractures
- Severe burns
- Acute allergic reactions or asthma attacks

If your emergency is life-threatening, your initial emergency-room care and your ambulance service will be covered, although you may have to pay a copayment, especially if you are not admitted to the hospital. You or someone acting on your behalf should notify your HMO doctor's office or your HMO about your emergency care as soon as possible; most HMOs require notification within twenty-four to forty-eight hours. Your HMO will want to take responsibility for your follow-up care and may even want to transfer you to another hospital once you are medically stable. The hospital that provides your emergency care may require you to pay the bill before you leave. If that happens, make sure you receive an itemized copy of the bill and your treatment record. Immediately contact your HMO's member service or claims department to find out how to get reimbursed.

## Handling an Emergency

HMO rules on what to do in an emergency can cause serious confusion, anxiety, and dissatisfaction for members, and they are a common reason for disputes between HMOs and members over whether care should be covered. Because emergencies are never foreseeable, you should take the time now to understand what to do when an emergency arises.

The examples that have been used to help you tell the difference between the kinds of emergencies for which you should call first and those for which you don't have to call first may seem pretty straightforward, at least on paper. But when you are faced with blood or extreme pain or fear, especially if it is your child's or another loved one's, you may find it very difficult to follow the rules. Your natural reaction may be to call an ambulance or the police for help. You are reacting to symptoms, and to you they look life-threatening. But your HMO is going to react to the diagnosis. If it turns out that the situation was not that serious and that you could have called first, emergency coverage may be denied. Here are some tips on emergency care that should help you get the care you need and avoid problems with your coverage.

▶Make a good-faith effort to call your HMO if you possibly can before you go to an emergency room, even if you are frightened. You may get some immediate medical advice that will help prevent a worse problem.

▶If you aren't sure how serious the emergency is and you call your HMO or HMO doctor, but you don't get an immediate response from someone who can give you medical advice, make note of the time and phone number you called, leave a message that you are going to the hospital (tell which one), and say you will have the hospital contact the HMO when you get there.

▶If you go to a hospital emergency room, and by the time you get there the situation seems to be less serious, call your HMO or have the emergency room staff call your HMO before you are evaluated or treated.

You might also want to ask your primary care clinician at your first appointment for any specific advice he or she has on how to handle emergencies.

## Preparing for an Emergency

Even if you are familiar with your HMO's rules, it's hard to be calm and rational when a medical emergency occurs. There also may be times when you could lose control over the decisions that are made about your medical care, for instance if the police, fire department, or an ambulance responds, or a friend or family member tries to help. The more prepared you are, the better the chance you'll get the care you need and that it will be covered by your HMO. Here are some tips to get you ready for an emergency:

◆ Make sure you know what number to call (911 or your community's seven-digit emergency number) in a life-threatening emergency.

◆ Know how to get to the hospital emergency room closest to your home, and how to give directions to someone else who may be driving.

◆ Know what number to call to reach your HMO or HMO doctor for instructions in a less serious emergency. Will you be able to speak with someone who can give you immediate medical advice? If not, how quickly will the HMO be able to reach someone who can? Does it depend on the time of day or night?

◆ Carry your HMO membership card with you at all times and make sure there are emergency instructions and an emergency phone number on it. Write the number down if it isn't there.

◆ Know who to notify at your HMO if you receive medical care in a life-threatening emergency, and how soon notification of your HMO is required.

◆ If you have a child at school or camp, make sure the school or camp nurse has a copy of your child's HMO membership card, information about special medical needs such as medications, and the details of your child's health coverage, including what to do in an emergency.

◆ If you are being cared for by someone who is not a member of your HMO, make sure he or she knows what to do if you have a medical emergency (for instance, children taking care of their elderly parents).

CASE EXAMPLE:
WHEN IS A MEDICAL CRISIS AN EMERGENCY?

*John loves to watch his daughter Carey play baseball. She's still learning the fundamentals, but she was chosen to play catcher because she has a good arm and always hustles. After every game, she looks as if she spent half her time diving into the dirt to block wild pitches. Today, Carey's enthusiasm got the best of her. Chasing a foul ball, she ran into the other team's dugout, fell down the steps, and landed hard, face down. When John reached the scene, her face was covered with blood and it looked as if she had a nasty gash on her scalp. Not only that, but John was afraid she might have landed on her arm and broken it. Someone yelled, "Call an ambulance," and her manager ran to a pay phone to call 911 for help. John remembered that his HMO required him to call them first unless an emergency was life-threatening, but his main concern was getting help for his daughter, and he wasn't about to overrule her manager. What should John do?*

*This situation was doubly difficult for him: first, because his daughter appeared to be badly hurt and was obviously scared and in pain, and second, because her manager felt responsible for taking control of the situation. And while he knew that Carey's injury was not life-threatening, she had hit her head, so a serious injury was a possibility.*

*Wanting to make a good-faith effort to reach his HMO, John gave another parent his HMO membership card and asked him to call the emergency number on the front, tell them what had happened, and tell them John would call again from the hospital. He knew that emergency calls were recorded, so his effort to follow the rules as well as he could under the circumstances would be documented. The ambulance the manager had called came and took Carey and John to the hospital, where his wife was waiting for them. She immediately made two calls, to their HMO and to Carey's pediatrician, to let them know what was happening.*

*Carey's head cut was stitched up in the hospital's outpatient clinic, her teeth and arm were checked and found to be okay, and she was sent home. John made a follow-up call to Carey's pediatrician, who had already been in touch with the hospital clinic. Later, he paid his HMO's $50 emergency copayment. (If Carey had been hospitalized, he wouldn't have had to pay it.) Other than that, he never saw a bill.*

# HMO COVERAGE
# WHEN YOU'RE AWAY FROM HOME

Hardly anyone spends all of his or her time at home, so it is important to know what is covered and what you should do to get medical care when you are away from your HMO's service area. It's also important to know how your HMO defines its service area so you will know when you are outside of it. (This is commonly referred to as being "out of area.") With HMOs expanding and merging, this may not be so easy to figure out. For instance, a Boston, Massachusetts, HMO member might discover that she is still "in area" when vacationing in the White Mountains of New Hampshire. The information you need should be in your member contract. If you're not sure, check with your HMO's member service department.

All HMOs cover serious or life-threatening emergencies when you are outside their service area in the same way they do when you are in area. You don't have to call in advance for authorization if taking the time to do so would endanger your life or cause serious impairment or disability.

Most, but not all, HMOs allow you to get urgent care when you are out of area without calling for authorization in advance. One common definition for covered out-of-area urgent care is the "medically necessary treatment for the sudden onset of any unforeseeable illness or injury." This might include a sprain or broken bone, a minor cut requiring stitches, or a severe earache.

If you are hospitalized out of area, you will have to notify your HMO doctor or HMO, usually within forty-eight hours. Your HMO will probably require you to have any nonhospital follow-up care provided or authorized by your HMO doctor. If you have to be hospitalized for a long time, the HMO may arrange to have you moved from an out-of-area hospital back to one of its affiliated hospitals.

Most HMOs do not cover you out of area for preventive care (such as a physical exam, Pap test, or vaccination); for care you could have foreseen or anticipated before leaving home (such as the removal of a cast, blood-pressure monitoring, elective surgery, or a full-term or near-full-term childbirth); or for follow-up care that could be safely delayed until you return to the care of your HMO doctor (such as physical therapy).

Note: Different rules may apply for students who are attending school outside their HMO's service area. Some HMOs cover students for types of care that would not normally be covered for nonstudent members who are out of area.

The way HMOs apply these general rules can vary greatly, so make sure you understand what you must do to be covered out of area. Here are some key issues to consider:

◆ How does your HMO define "out of area"? Is it based on a list of cities and towns that are "in area," or do you also have to be a certain distance from home, or from an HMO doctor's office or clinic, to be out of area?

◆ Since HMO service areas can be confusing and they can change over time, call your HMO before you travel or go on vacation and ask whether you will be in area or out of area.

◆ Does your HMO have different rules that apply when you are out of the country? For instance, are you required to call your HMO before getting care when you are in the United States but not when you are abroad?

◆ Are you covered if you get care for a medical problem that is unexpected but not urgent, such as the flu? If so, do you have to call first for authorization?

◆ Are you covered for urgent care, and if so, do you have to call first for authorization? Some HMOs have 800 numbers or they ask you to call collect.

◆ Can you see any doctor (primary care or specialist), or go to any clinic or hospital clinic when you need emergency or urgent care out of area, or are there restrictions?

◆ Does your HMO have an arrangement with HMOs in other parts of the country to provide you with care when you are traveling in their enrollment areas? Do you have to use these other HMOs, or is it your choice?

◆ If you have prescription drug coverage with your HMO, are you also covered for prescriptions written and/or filled out of area?

◆ How soon do you have to notify your HMO if you are hospitalized out of area, and how will your follow-up care be handled?

◆ What will you have to do to get paid back by your HMO if you receive out-of-area medical care that is covered, but the doctor or hospital makes you pay for it?

◆ Does your HMO have different out-of-area coverage rules for students who are away at school? Do you have to sign up for any special program for student out-of-area coverage?

◆ What about children who are away at camp? How will the camp know what they should do to make sure any care your child needs is covered?

## MEDICAL CARE FROM SPECIALISTS

Your HMO primary care doctor or a member of his or her clinical team (a nurse practitioner or physician's assistant) will be able to take care of most of your medical needs. There are times, however, when you will need care from a specialist for the diagnosis or treatment of your medical problems. If you want that care to be covered fully by your HMO, you must have authorization in advance and a referral to the specialist. Some types of HMOs allow you to arrange your own specialty care, either inside or outside the HMO network, but you'll pay more for that option.

Specialties that require a referral from your HMO primary care doctor or your HMO could include: allergy, audiology, cardiology, chiropractic, dermatology, ENT (ear, nose, and throat), endocrinology, fertility and endocrinology, gastroenterology, genetics, gynecology, hematology, infectious disease, mental health, nephrology, neurology, nutrition, obstetrics, occupational therapy, oncology, ophthalmology, optometry, orthopedics, pain therapy, physical therapy, podiatry, pulmonary, radiology, and other diagnostic services, rheumatology, speech and language pathology, substance abuse, surgery, and urology.

HMOs may have some of these specialists "in house," meaning they are located in the HMOs' health centers, clinics, or group practices. They may have "preferred" or "participating" specialists who are part of the HMO network. Or they may refer patients to specialists outside their network, sometimes in other states or regions, for very rare conditions. Different referral rules may apply to each type of specialist.

Most HMOs allow you to seek care from a few types of specialists without prior authorization and a referral, but you should always check first if you are not sure, otherwise you may have to pay the bill for your care.

## How to Get a Referral

If you think you need specialty care, you should immediately discuss it with your primary care doctor, either in person or by phone. Referrals must almost always be authorized before you get HMO specialty care. Typically a referral form must be filled out by your primary care doctor and approved by your HMO. Referral forms specify who the authorized specialist is; what the specialist is expected to do; how long the referral is good for (you may be required to schedule your appointment within thirty to sixty days or else get a new referral); and the number of covered visits. In other words, they are not open-ended.

If your doctor recommends a referral, you should be given a clear reason for the referral, what you should expect, and what role he or she will play in coordinating or following up on your specialty care. Sometimes, your doctor or your HMO will deny a referral request as unnecessary or inappropriate. If that happens, your doctor should be able to tell you why it was denied, and help you with an alternative course of diagnosis or treatment. If you have a particular specialist in mind, you should discuss your preference with your primary care doctor to see if a referral is appropriate and possible.

If you are told by your primary care doctor that specialty care has been authorized, you should still confirm your referral when you call to make an appointment with the specialist. You don't want to show up for your appointment and find out that the paperwork has not been completed. If you feel that you are being denied access to specialty care that you need, you should immediately bring your concern to the attention of your primary care doctor or talk to your HMO's member service department. Here are some key issues to consider:

◆ Does your HMO allow you to refer yourself to any types of specialists without prior authorization from

your primary care doctor? Under any special circumstances?

◆ Do you know, step by step, how to get a referral for specialty care?

◆ If your primary care doctor has to make a referral, will
you have more than one specialist to choose from? If so,
will your doctor help you with the decision?

◆ Are there particular referral specialists you want to
have care for you; if so, how will you let your primary
care doctor know your wishes?

◆ Are there any types of specialists whose services are
specifically excluded from your HMO's benefits (chiropractors, for instance)?

◆ Are there any limits on referrals in terms of who and
what they cover, and for how long? How do you extend or
renew a referral?

◆ If you get a bill from a specialist for services that are
authorized and covered by your HMO, do you know what
to do?

CASE EXAMPLE:
WHEN YOU WANT THE BEST SPECIALTY CARE

*When Khalid found an HMO that offered direct non-
group membership, he was delighted. He had been very
healthy all his life, so there were no restrictions on his
coverage, and the HMO was $100 a month less expensive
than a traditional insurance plan he looked into. Still,
his monthly premium was high, and he had to pay it all
himself. In three years of membership, he had gone to his
HMO doctor only a few times, so he was starting to won-
der if he was getting his money's worth. It didn't help*

*that a friend kept telling him, "Just wait until you're
really sick. Your doctor's not going to want to take care of
you because the cost comes out of his pocket."*

*Then, during a routine checkup, his doctor detected a
possible heart problem. He told Khalid that he would
arrange to have him referred to a cardiologist who
belonged to the same group practice. A few days after his
first appointment with the cardiologist, Khalid received
a phone call telling him he was going to be referred to
another cardiologist instead: one who practiced at a hospital an hour away. Not only was Khalid scared about
his heart problem, he was convinced that his friend had
been right: his doctor and his cardiologist partner were
trying to pass off his case to another specialist so the cost
of his care wouldn't come out of their pockets. Or maybe
his HMO had chosen the other cardiologist to take care
of him because she would charge less. Khalid was very
anxious. What should he do?*

*A common concern HMO members have, especially
those who were somewhat reluctant to join an HMO or
who didn't have a clear understanding of how they work,
is that medical decisions will be made primarily on the
basis of cost. This reinforces the idea that "HMOs are
great until you get really sick." In fact, many independent studies have shown that HMOs provide care that is
just as good as traditional fee-for-service medicine. But
when you feel awful or are afraid that something is very
wrong, that's when a recommendation by your HMO doctor for a less expensive course of diagnosis or treatment
may worry you.*

*In Khalid's case, a big problem was the lack of com-
munication between his primary care doctor and himself, which fed his suspicions. He needed to ask "why?"
every step of the way: asking for a full explanation of*

*what his problem might be, how it would be diagnosed, and what the treatment options were. His primary care doctor should have explained the medical reasons for his first referral and the new referral, and answered his concerns about whether cost was a factor.*

*Khalid decided to call his HMO's member service department to voice his concerns. The next morning he was called back by his primary care doctor, who apologized and explained that the reason for the second referral was that the second cardiologist had more experience with Khalid's kind of heart problem. His doctor then arranged a phone call between Khalid and the cardiologist, so they could go over some of Khalid's questions and concerns. After it was over, Khalid felt like a much more active participant in the decision making about his care.*

---

## Phone Tips for New Members

By now, it should be clear how important it is to call your HMO or your HMO doctor when you have a medical problem or a question about your care. Here are some things to keep in mind when you call:

- If you have a medical emergency, say, "This is a medical emergency. I need help right away."
- Identify yourself as a new member of the HMO when you tell your name.
- If you have chosen a primary care doctor, give the doctor's name; if not, say so.
- If possible, have your membership card (or those of other members for whom you are calling) ready in case you are asked for information that might be on the card.
- If you or a family member needs immediate attention because you are sick, say so, and be ready to explain exactly what is wrong: symptoms, temperature, how long

the patient has been sick, changes in how the patient looks or feels, and any information about the patient's allergies, previous conditions, or medications.

- If there is other information you need as a new member, make a list of questions before you call. If you are confused, keep asking.
- If you aren't sure where your doctor's office is located, how to get there, or what days and hours it is open, ask during your first call, and write the information down.
- Also ask if there is a special number you should call if you need urgent care at a time when your doctor's office is closed.

The busiest times for most doctors and HMOs are on Mondays and the days after holidays, and for the first few hours of the day, so if you don't have an urgent need for help, try calling at another time. If you want a same-day appointment, call as early in the day as possible.

If you have to cancel an appointment, try to call at least twenty-four hours in advance. If you fail to call in advance, your HMO may charge you a fee for the appointment because the time could have been given to someone else who needed it.

## GETTING HMO HOSPITAL CARE

As with most specialty care, hospital care must be authorized in advance by your HMO primary care doctor or your HMO, whether it is for inpatient care (you occupy a hospital bed overnight) or outpatient care (you don't occupy a hospital bed overnight). The only exceptions are life-threatening emergencies or when you are outside your HMO's service area. This is true even if your hospitalization is ordered by a specialist to whom you have been referred.

HMOs want to keep you out of the hospital when possible; they want you to go to an appropriate hospital; and they want your stay to be as short as possible. At the same time, HMOs shouldn't want your stay to be shorter than medically necessary, because that could lead to further medical problems and additional cost. Your condition could worsen or you might even have to be readmitted to the hospital.

Popular ideas about hospitalization have changed dramatically over the past several decades, and hospital stays have become shorter and shorter. Procedures that used to be done in a hospital to prepare a patient for surgery can now be done in a doctor's office. Medical technology allows doctors to perform many surgeries on an outpatient basis in a hospital or "surgi-center." Recovery times are much shorter, because of new technology and procedures and because experts now agree that getting patients back on their feet as soon as medically appropriate is better for them. Postoperative care and rehabilitation can often be provided in the home or in other nonhospital settings. Hospitals are no longer seen as the best places for "rest and recuperation." Since hospital stays are shorter, good communication among doctors and other clinicians, patients, and the HMO is especially important.

Some HMOs operate their own hospitals. Some have preferred hospitals in their network. With others, the hospital you go to will depend on where your HMO doctor has admitting privileges. When hospitalization is recommended, your HMO doctor and HMO should be very much involved, before, during, and after you are admitted. You may encounter one or more of the following:

►Utilization review: Your doctor's decision to hospitalize you will be reviewed, and approved or denied, by a medical professional employed by, or under contract to, your HMO. Utilization review may also be used to determine how long you should be hospitalized.

►Preadmission certification: You will need formal authorization before you can be admitted to the hospital.

►Utilization management or case management: A team of medical professionals employed by or under contract to your HMO will work with your HMO doctor and the hospital to plan your admission, review your care, and plan for your discharge.

►Discharge planning: A team of nurses or other medical professionals will work with you and your family, the hospital, and outside medical resources like home care or skilled nursing, to try to keep your hospital stay to a minimum and make sure continuing care is available in another setting if it is needed.

Most HMOs have very comprehensive coverage for hospitalization and understand how important it is to manage hospital care well, for both cost and quality. If you follow the basic rule—get authorization from your HMO doctor or HMO before you are hospitalized, except in the case of a life-threatening emergency—nothing should stand in the way of your receiving the kind of care you need.

One common concern among HMO members is that they will have to wait too long for "elective" procedures. You will certainly wait longer for hospital care that is not urgently needed. But how long is too long? As with specialty care, if you feel that you are being denied access to needed hospital care, take your concerns immediately to your HMO doctor or your HMO's member service department.

Here are some key issues to consider about your HMO hospital care:

◆ Do you know what hospital you would be admitted to for routine (secondary) care; for specialized (tertiary) care? How much choice do you have?

◆ Do you know how to get hospital care authorized, and how to get a second opinion or file an appeal if authorization is denied?

◆ If you are hospitalized, what role will your primary care doctor play before, during, and after your hospital stay?

◆ How will decisions be made about how long you will stay in the hospital, and to what extent will you be involved in those decisions?

◆ What resources will be available to you when you leave the hospital to aid in your recovery or for additional treatment, and will they be covered by your HMO?

◆ Does your HMO require a copayment for hospitalization; under what circumstances?

◆ Are there any hospital services that are limited in coverage or not covered at all (e.g., private rooms, televisions, prescription medications)?

◆ If you receive a bill from a hospital for services that are authorized and covered by your HMO, do you know what to do?

◆ If you are a Medicare HMO member, is there anything special you need to know about your hospital care or coverage?

CASE EXAMPLE:
WHEN YOUR HOSPITAL STAY SEEMS TOO SHORT

*When George entered the hospital for his operation, he was apprehensive but prepared. His HMO primary care physician had authorized and made the arrangements for his hospitalization, and had performed a series of preoperative tests in his office. George had received information from the hospital in the mail, telling him all about check-in procedures, rules for visitors, and even what kind of food to expect. He knew he wouldn't be facing any bills from the hospital, except for the extra cost of a private room and any videotapes he rented during his stay, because those aren't covered by his HMO.*

*On the morning of George's operation, his surgeon had come by to talk with him, and had indicated that he expected George to be in the hospital for four to five days. The operation went smoothly, and George began his recovery. On the evening of the second day, a nurse case manager from his HMO arrived to give him some "good news." He would be going home the next morning. George was shocked! He was still in pain, he was still hooked up to an intravenous tube, and he assumed that he needed four to five days in the hospital, just as his surgeon had said, before it was safe for him to go home. What should George do?*

*George was the victim of several kinds of miscommunication, and it wouldn't be surprising if he concluded that his HMO was pushing him out of the hospital to save money.*

*Ideally, George should have had an opportunity to meet with his HMO's nurse case manager and his surgeon before his operation to discuss how his discharge would be planned. He probably would have been told that his HMO encourages short hospital stays for good medical, as well as financial, reasons. Instead of being given an arbitrary estimate of his stay, he would have learned that his condition would be evaluated day to day, and that when certain medical criteria were met, he would be considered for discharge. A thorough discharge plan should have been created for him, and it should have been written into his hospital chart. His HMO primary care doctor should have followed his case, kept in*

*touch with the hospital specialist, and worked with
George and the HMO nurse case manager to make sure
any necessary follow-up care was in place.*

*George decided to call his primary care doctor's office,
and, for good measure, his HMO's member service
department. In the early evening, he was visited by his
HMO's nurse case manager, who explained to George
and his wife the medical criteria that were being used to
evaluate his readiness to leave the hospital. While George
wasn't particularly happy, he felt somewhat reassured
that, from a medical point of view, he was ready to go
home. By morning, his primary care doctor had scheduled a follow-up appointment and arrangements had
been made for a home care nurse to help with home medical equipment George would need to use during his
recovery.*

## SKILLED NURSING
## AND REHABILITATIVE CARE

One way HMOs can help you get out of the hospital sooner
after a serious illness or operation is by providing you with
skilled nursing care or rehabilitative care, either at your
home or in a skilled nursing ("extended care") facility or
rehabilitation hospital. Skilled nursing and rehabilitative
care must be authorized in advance by your HMO and delivered by providers who participate in, or are approved by,
your HMO. There may be limits on the total number of days
of skilled nursing and rehabilitative care your HMO will
cover each year. HMOs don't cover long-term or custodial
nursing-home care unless it is a special added benefit.
(Custodial care means services that are furnished mainly to
help a disabled or infirm person with activities of daily living, like dressing, feeding, and personal hygiene.)

# HOME HEALTH CARE

Many types of treatment can now be provided just as effectively, and for less money, at your home. In addition to providing skilled nursing, HMOs cover other types of home health care when they are authorized by your HMO doctor or your HMO and delivered by approved providers. Many HMOs, for example, either encourage or expect women to leave the hospital one day after normal childbirth, or three days after a cesarean section. The HMO then provides some type of follow-up care for both mother and baby at home.

Covered home health care services may include physical therapy, occupational therapy, speech therapy, nutrition counseling, intravenous (IV) therapy, durable medical equipment and supplies, medical social services, and the services of a home health aide. Meals, personal comfort items, and housekeeping services are usually not covered, and home services for custodial care are usually not covered.

# HOSPICE CARE

For patients who are terminally ill and are nearing the end of their lives, the most appropriate care may be hospice care. Hospice care focuses on keeping patients comfortable and helping them die in the most gentle and dignified way possible, rather than on trying to cure or reverse their illnesses (with surgery or radiation therapy, for example). Care for the dying can be provided in a hospice, in a hospital, or at home. The services, facilities, and staffs of hospice programs may be regulated and licensed by the state in order to ensure that the goals of comfort, quality, and dignity are achieved.

You should be able to find out if your HMO covers hospice care by looking in your member contract, especially if your state requires hospice care coverage. If you can't find a spe-

cific reference to hospice care in your contract, ask your
HMO doctor or your HMO's member service department.

If hospice care is a covered benefit, it will have to be
arranged or authorized by the patient's HMO doctor or
HMO. There may be certain requirements for admission to a
hospice program, such as a diagnosis of an illness for which
the life expectancy is six months or less, and for which "pal-
liative care" (pain control and relief of symptoms) rather
than "curative care" is most appropriate.

Hospice care benefits may be limited to a maximum number of days of care. It will be important for you to understand
what specific services are covered, such as drugs, oxygen,
medical equipment and supplies, nursing or social worker
care, homemaker services, nutritional counseling, and food
supplements. In some states, covered hospice services also
include a fixed number of counseling sessions for the family
of the patient, either before or after the patient's death.

## COVERAGE FOR PRESCRIPTION DRUGS

For most HMO members, prescription drug coverage is a big
money-saver when it comes to out-of-pocket costs, but it also
means higher premiums. If you have joined an HMO
through your employer, the company will decide whether or
not you have prescription drug coverage as part of your benefits plan. Some smaller employers don't include it because
of the added cost, and some HMOs offer low-cost Medicare
plans without drug coverage, but the vast majority of HMO
members have it. Since prescription drugs play such an
important role in health care today, and because drugs can
be so expensive, people without drug coverage may find the
quality of their care limited by what they can afford to pay
out of pocket if they become seriously ill.

If you have HMO prescription drug coverage you will have
to make only a moderate copayment for each medication pre-

scribed (usually up to a thirty-day supply for each prescription). To control their costs, most HMOs limit their coverage to a network of participating pharmacies, and they cover only prescriptions written by an HMO doctor (or other HMO clinician, like a nurse practitioner or physician's assistant, if it is allowed by state law). The participating pharmacies may be located in your HMO's health centers or clinics, or they may include local community pharmacies, chain pharmacies, or some combination of all three. If you are not sure which pharmacies are in your HMO's network, call your HMO to find out the names and locations of those most convenient for you.

Your HMO may have a mail-order prescription drug program for people who take the same drugs over a long period of time. In some HMOs, mail order is optional for your convenience; in others it is required or strongly encouraged for maintenance medications. For instance, if you need a prescription for a thirty- to ninety-day supply, you may have to use the HMO's mail-order service.

Your HMO may also have a limited "formulary," that is, a list of drugs they consider to be most appropriate because they are the least expensive of several drugs that offer equivalent effectiveness in treating a given condition. If your HMO requires its physicians and participating pharmacies to prescribe from their formulary, it's possible that a medication you have been taking will not be on the formulary list, and you will have to switch.

Your HMO may also require or encourage the use of generic drugs. Federal laws set the same standards of strength, quality, purity, and effectiveness for all medications, whether brand name or generic. What may vary is the size, shape, strength, coating, taste (for liquids), inactive ingredients, packaging, and price. Some of these factors may affect your body's reaction to certain medications, so discuss this with your clinician or pharmacist.

If you have any questions or concerns about whether the medication you are offered by your HMO is as effective or safe as the one you've been taking, talk to your HMO primary care doctor or pharmacist.

Also, remember that most HMOs cover only "medically necessary" prescription drugs and, sometimes, medically necessary nonprescription drugs and medical supplies. Oral contraceptives and some birth control devices like diaphragms may be covered, along with syringes and blood- and urine-testing products for the treatment of diabetes and some nonprescription nutritional products. Drugs that are experimental or unproven are usually not covered, nor are drugs that are for cosmetic purposes, such as skin- and hair-restoration products. Antismoking medications, such as nicotine gum and nicotine patches, are sometimes covered, but you may be required to attend a smoking-cessation class at the same time.

If you have prescription drug coverage, make sure you know what is and is not covered, and whether you pay a percentage of drug costs or a fixed fee per prescription. There should be a limit on how much you will have to pay out of pocket each year. If that is the case, make sure you keep track of your payments. When you reach your dollar limit, your HMO will pay 100 percent of the cost of covered drugs.

---

## Using Prescription Drugs Wisely

It is important to your good health for you to understand what drug you are taking, why you are taking it, and what if any precautions or special instructions you need to follow. Your best source of this information is your doctor or pharmacist. For instance, you should know:

- What are the expected results of your medication? How long does it take to begin working?
- How long and how often will you need to take the medicine?

- How much do you take each time you take it?
- Do you take it with water? with food? with juice?
- What do you do if you miss a dose by mistake?
- What foods, drinks, or other medications (prescription or over-the-counter) should you avoid while you are taking your prescription medication?
- What restrictions on activities should you observe, such as driving a car or operating other machinery?
- What common side effects can be expected and what can you do to minimize them?
- What uncommon and potentially serious side effects could be experienced, and what can you do to avoid them?
- What is the expiration date and what should you do then?
- Are there lifestyle changes you can make that will help you avoid the need for medication?

## POTENTIAL PROBLEM AREAS

There are some conditions that can get very confusing and frustrating for HMO members. Dental care, vision care, hearing care, cosmetic surgery, alternative therapies, and medical equipment are all areas where there is a fine line between what is considered medically necessary (and therefore covered by your HMO) and what is not considered medically necessary (and therefore not covered).

### Dental, Vision, and Hearing Care

Standard HMOs limit coverage for dental, vision, and hearing care to what is considered medically necessary. Some HMOs also offer special plans or "riders" that can be bought separately by employers for their employees. These separate plans offer much more comprehensive coverage for people who are willing to use the HMO's network of dental and vision care providers.

Most standard HMO plans divide dental, vision, and hearing care into three categories:

◆ Medically necessary care that involves your mouth, teeth, eyes, or ears, which is covered as long as you follow the rules that apply to other kinds of medical care.

◆ Preventive care, such as routine teeth cleaning and examinations or routine vision and hearing exams. You may find that there are limitations on how many preventive care visits are covered each year, and preventive dental coverage may be limited to children.

◆ Care that is not medically necessary, including dental braces and other orthodontia, tooth bonding, dentures, corrective lenses, and hearing aids, which is not covered unless it results from treatment of a medical condition.

Since there is a very fine line between medically necessary care and nonmedical care when it comes to the mouth, teeth, eyes, and ears, patients and HMOs can easily disagree about coverage. For instance, if you are hit in the mouth with a baseball bat, emergency care of your teeth and gums would probably be covered, but not restoration of your teeth or follow-up care. The removal of wisdom teeth may not be covered unless they are impacted *and* infected. Contact lenses are not covered unless they replace your eyes' natural lenses during surgery for cataracts or some other eye disease. Hearing care may be covered if you suffer an injury or disease of your ears, but hearing aids are not.

## TMJ: Painful and Confusing

A condition that seems to lead to frequent complaints about coverage is Temporomandibular Joint (TMJ) disorder. Your TMJ, or jaw joint, is situated directly in front of your ear. TMJ disorders occur when the joints, jaw, and muscles don't work together correctly, and you experience symptoms like headaches, facial pain and stiffness, and noises in the ear. Diagnosis of TMJ is usually covered by HMOs, but coverage of treatment is not so clear cut because there are several options. TMJ can be treated with nonsurgical therapies and appliances, including plastic splints and dental treatments that are not covered by most HMOs. If dental care doesn't work, or if the condition is diagnosed as a medical problem, surgery might be required, and surgery probably will be covered. Someone who is suffering from acute TMJ pain might be unwilling to wait to see if nonsurgical treatments will work, especially if the HMO doesn't cover them. The best course of action is to make sure you understand your HMO's rules for coverage of TMJ disorders, and seek both medical and dental advice from your HMO.

## Cosmetic Surgery

Cosmetic or plastic surgery, which is any medical procedure to change or restore appearance, is covered only under very limited circumstances by most HMOs. For instance, when cosmetic surgery or reconstructive surgery is needed to repair serious damage or disfigurement from an injury or illness, it is covered. When cosmetic surgery is intended to repair severe disfigurement from a birth defect or anomaly, it will probably be covered, but coverage for some conditions may apply only to people who were members of the HMO at the time of their birth. When it is intended to improve a person's appearance, whether or not the member's mental or emotional outlook would also be improved, cosmetic surgery is not covered.

Some types of cosmetic surgery are almost never covered, like face lifts, liposuction, breast enlargement, treatment of acne scars, and removal of tattoos. Others raise tough questions that you will need to discuss with your HMO doctor or HMO if you think they apply to you or a member of your family. For instance, is breast reduction covered if a woman is suffering from serious discomfort; when does discomfort become a medical problem that makes breast reduction medically necessary? How severe does a birth defect or anomaly have to be in order for cosmetic surgery to be covered; does it have to interfere with a person's physical functioning, or is there a different standard? Is removal of a growth on the skin covered, or does it have to be cancerous?

If you disagree with your HMO on coverage of a certain type of cosmetic surgery, seek a second opinion or file an appeal of their coverage decision. Don't have the surgery done without authorization in advance unless you are willing to take the chance that you will have to pay for it.

## Alternative Therapies

A study published in the *New England Journal of Medicine* in 1993 found that nearly one in three American adults uses "unconventional" or alternative therapies for the treatment of serious medical conditions. Many of these alternative therapies are viewed by people trained in traditional Western medicine as ineffective, and in some cases nothing more than quackery. Other therapies, like acupuncture, chiropractic, yoga, meditation, polarity, biofeedback, homeopathy, and nutritional therapies are considered beneficial, and may be covered by some health insurers and HMOs. If nothing else, much of the medical community now agrees that there is an important relationship between the mind and body, and views alternative therapies as a way to treat the "whole person."

What is missing with most alternative therapies is scientific evidence of what works and what doesn't work, and under what conditions. Until that evidence is developed in controlled experimental trials and accepted by the medical community at large, HMOs and other health insurers will continue to categorize most alternative therapies as "unproven."

So while some HMO doctors will accept the idea that alternative therapies should be an important part of their treatment approach, and they may be willing to refer you to a nonmedical practitioner for treatment, you will need to check with your HMO in advance to find out if you are covered. If you are interested in alternative therapies, ask your HMO if it ever covers them, and what you would have to do to be covered.

## Medical Equipment

In the course of an illness, or following an accident, you may need to use medical equipment. Medical equipment must be recommended or prescribed by your HMO doctor in order to be covered. There are two general categories of covered equipment: durable medical equipment, like wheelchairs, crutches, canes, walkers, oxygen equipment, and hospital beds; and corrective appliances or prosthetic equipment, like artificial limbs and eyes, back, leg, and neck braces, and ostomy supplies. You will probably find that your HMO's contract includes a long list of equipment, ranging from air conditioners to arch supports to exercise bicycles, that is not covered because it is not considered medically necessary. As mentioned earlier, hearing aids, eyeglasses and contact lenses, and dental appliances are usually not covered. If your contract is unclear about what is covered, ask your HMO's member service department. You will also want to know whether your HMO will pay for the fitting, repair, adjustment, or replacement of covered equipment, and how often.

For medical equipment that is covered by your HMO, you may have to pay part of the cost of equipment (20 to 50 percent is typical) or there may also be a maximum amount your HMO will pay toward your medical equipment in a year ($1500 per year, for example).

Remember, even if a procedure or medical device is recommended to you by your HMO doctor, that isn't an absolute guarantee that it will be covered. Your HMO contract governs your benefits, and it is up to you to make sure you understand them, and their limitations, before you get care that may fall into one of these problem areas.

## OTHER IMPORTANT BENEFITS ISSUES

The benefits issues discussed in this chapter have been primarily focused on getting coverage for the health care you need. There are other areas covered in your HMO contract that are also very important to your membership, especially those that involve the terms of your relationship with your HMO and ways it could change over time.

### Termination of Your Membership

Your member contract will describe in detail the circumstances under which you and/or your dependents could have your membership contract terminated. For instance:

◆ If you lose your job, resign, or retire from the company through which you are covered.

◆ If you or your employer fails to pay the premium.

◆ If your HMO requires that you and other family members live in their enrollment or service area for all or most of the year and you do not.

◆ If the subscriber provided false or misleading information on the application, or if a member commits fraud.

As mentioned above, dependents can also lose their coverage if they no longer meet the HMO's eligibility requirements, for instance, a dependent child who marries or reaches the cutoff age.

If your employer gets into financial trouble and fails to pay your premiums, you may find yourself without coverage through no fault or choice of your own. Your termination could be retroactive to the time your employer last paid your premiums, in which case you may be asked to pay for care you have already received because it was not covered.

With most HMOs, your membership will end when you become eligible for Medicare, unless you enroll in Medicare and your HMO offers a Medicare plan that supplements your Medicare coverage.

The issue of termination is described in detail in your HMO contract. Obviously, losing coverage can be devastating, especially if you are in the middle of treatment for a serious medical problem. The good news is that you have certain rights that will help protect you from losing coverage altogether. The bad news is that your so-called "conversion" options may be very expensive, since they will require you to pay your entire premium.

## How to Stay Covered

Unless your contract is terminated because of fraud or some illegal act on your part, your HMO is obligated to provide you with adequate notice and the opportunity to continue your coverage in some fashion. If you can afford it, you should take advantage of one of these "conversion" options right away. Otherwise you may be without coverage for a longer time, and you will find that it is more difficult to get new coverage that will meet your needs, especially if you have a preexisting medical problem. If your coverage can be continued without interruption, you may not be faced with preexisting-condition restrictions. The most common conversion options are as follows:

▶HMO members who lose their employer group eligibility or their eligibility as dependents may be able to continue their group coverage under certain state or federal laws. (The best known is called COBRA.) If your membership ends because of layoff, a reduction in your work hours, your resignation, or your loss of dependent status because of the age, divorce, legal separation, or death of the subscriber, contact the subscriber's employer for information on your options. If you are allowed to continue your coverage, it will probably be for a limited amount of time, and you will have to pay the full premium to the subscriber's employer.

▶Members who lose their employer group eligibility may also be able to convert to nongroup membership if they do so within a required amount of time. Nongroup members may not get the same benefits as group members, premiums will probably be higher, and you will be required to pay the full amount of the premium, either on a monthly or quarterly basis. But, as mentioned earlier, nongroup conversion will guarantee continuation of your coverage, and it should be available without any preexisting-condition restrictions.

▶It may be more difficult to convert to your HMO's nongroup coverage if your employer decided to drop your HMO, or if your group membership was terminated for fraud or other misconduct. And you will still be required to meet your HMO's other eligibility requirements, such as those regarding where you live or how old you are.

►If your HMO requires that you live within its enrollment or service area for all or most of the year, and you move out of the enrollment area, you may be offered the option to switch to another HMO or an insurance plan that has a special arrangement with your HMO, without having a break in your coverage. Your benefits and premiums will probably be different, and you will have to pay the full premium unless you have group coverage through your new plan.

►If you become eligible for Medicare and you want more coverage than your basic Medicare benefits, your HMO will be able to convert you to its Medicare plan, if it offers one. If it doesn't have a plan for Medicare beneficiaries, ask its member service department or your employer for information about plans that offer coverage to supplement Medicare.

## When Your Contract Changes

From time to time, most commonly on the anniversary date of your membership contract, your HMO may change your benefits. Benefit changes can take place because your employer wants to increase or cut back benefits; your HMO might make changes or offer new "products" with different benefits; or new state or federal laws might require benefit changes. Your employer or your HMO should notify you in advance of any benefit changes, and your HMO should send you an entirely new contract or amendments to your contract. In either case, you should read them carefully so that you understand any new rules affecting your care and coverage. Several common types of benefit changes are:

►Increased copayments: Your HMO might increase the amount you have to pay for office visits, prescription drugs, emergency room visits, or hospital stays.

►Changes in other kinds of cost sharing: Some HMOs require you to share the cost of benefits like medical equipment or mental health and substance-abuse treatment. "Point-of-service" plans require you to pay a deductible and coinsurance when you choose to get care outside your HMO's network.

►Changes in what is covered: Many states have passed laws that require HMOs and other health plans to cover specific types of treatment. Some recent examples include in vitro fertilization (IVF) and other infertility services, nutritional supplements, cardiac rehabilitation, hospice care, chiropractic, early intervention services for children, and bone-marrow transplantation for the treatment of advanced breast cancer. In most cases HMOs and insurers had excluded coverage for these treatments because they considered them to be experimental, unproven, or not medically necessary. Such new "mandated benefits" usually take effect within several months after the law requiring them is passed. Your HMO might choose to add benefits, either for procedures and treatments that are no longer considered experimental or because they make the HMO more attractive to consumers. An example of the former is coverage for organ transplantation, and of the latter, vision or dental benefits. On the other hand, your HMO could also cut back your benefits, for instance by restricting the number of routine physicals or mental health therapy sessions it will cover each year.

►Changes in the HMO's network: HMOs frequently change their networks of primary care doctors. An HMO might add doctors to make itself more accessible to more consumers, or drop doctors that don't meet its standards. It might also increase or reduce the number of facilities where members can receive certain types of hospital services or diagnostic tests. Selective networks usually result in lower costs for HMOs because they can direct more of their patients to particular hospitals or other medical providers in exchange for discounts. However, network changes can also have a serious impact on patients if existing medical relationships are disrupted. If such a change occurs, contact your HMO's member service department for help with your transition to a new provider. In response to selective HMO networks, some states have passed laws forcing HMOs to contract with certain types of health care providers, for example, chiropractors, acupuncturists, nurse midwives, or podiatrists. Another type of state mandate requires HMOs to include "any willing provider" in certain parts of their networks. For instance, HMOs might not be able to restrict their network of participating pharmacies for members who have prescription drug coverage. It is important to know whether a change in an HMO's network also means a change in its enrollment area. With an enrollment area change, some communities that used to be "out of area" could now be in area, requiring you to follow different rules if you are sick or injured.

▶Acquisitions and mergers: In some parts of the country, HMOs are buying one another or merging into single plans. Over time, this can have a huge impact on members, resulting in benefit and cost-sharing changes, new networks, new enrollment areas, and new eligibility requirements. Often, the biggest problem members face is confusion owing to poor communication. These changes seldom take place overnight, however, and if you have group coverage, your employer as well as your HMO should keep you informed about how they will affect you. Also, health plans going through acquisitions and mergers are especially sensitive to government regulators, so if you have any concerns or problems, you can contact the appropriate insurance or public health agency in your state.

## When Your Premium Changes

It is very likely that your HMO premium costs will change every year. You should expect to be told about premium changes in advance, by your HMO or your employer. If you have the option of switching plans, you should have plenty of time to consider doing so. If you are covered through your employer, your payroll deduction could change for two reasons: because your HMO premium goes up (or down), or because your employer changes its "contribution policy," the amount or percent it pays toward your HMO's total premium. Or both. If you pay the entire premium, these changes will affect you directly, dollar for dollar.

Why do premiums change from year to year? There are many causes, including hospital costs, clinical and administrative salaries and fees, drug and equipment costs, new technologies, new diseases, changes in administrative costs, general cost inflation in the economy, and so on. Also, HMOs try to make a profit each year, just like other businesses. If they are nonprofit HMOs, they try to end the year with "surpluses" that can be set aside to use for future investments or for protection against unexpected financial problems.

HMOs set their average premiums each year, based on how many members they expect to have enrolled, the mix of individual and family memberships, the expected average family size, how much it will cost to provide all of their care and coverage, and how much of a surplus they want to have at the end of the year. But no HMO charges everyone the same premium. Premium levels for the employees of each company or for other groupings (such as all nongroup members or all Medicare members) will depend to some degree on how much the HMO expects to spend to take care of them. If you are part of a high-cost group, your premiums may go up faster even if you are very healthy yourself. Competition also plays a role; your HMO may hold down your premiums because its competitors are less expensive.

One way or another, you are paying a lot for your HMO coverage, so you have the right to know why it costs what it does. If you think your premiums are too high, or rising too fast, talk to your employer or your HMO's member service department about it. And don't be satisfied with "Health care costs are going up everywhere." Ask for specifics about why your group's premiums have gone up, and what your HMO is doing to keep future premium increases down.

## Duplicate Coverage and Coordination of Benefits

There may be situations in which you are covered by more than one health plan contract or health insurance policy. You cannot, however, be covered or reimbursed for more than the cost of any care you receive. If you have duplicate coverage, you will be expected to work with your HMO to avoid duplication of your benefits. This is called "coordination of benefits."

Duplicate coverage can occur if you and your spouse both have health care coverage through your employers and you enroll each other and/or your dependent children in each other's health plans. Under certain circumstances, your medical care may be covered by motor vehicle insurance, home owners' insurance, personal injury insurance, workers' compensation, or government programs like Medicare, in addition to your HMO.

The general rule in the case of duplicate coverage is that one insurer is "primary" and the other plan or plans will be "secondary." First the primary plan pays its benefits, then the secondary plan pays. In some cases your HMO may be primary, in other cases it will be secondary. A complex set of rules decides which is which. If you let your HMO know about any additional coverage you have, it will be up to the HMO to coordinate benefits. It will tell you what steps you have to take to avoid duplicate payment and to make sure you don't get billed for covered care.

## Subrogation

What happens if someone else is legally responsible for causing your injury or illness? He or she may have insurance that will pay for all or part of your care. In that case, your HMO may choose to enforce its "subrogation" rights to recover the cost of any services it has provided for which another party is liable to pay. It can do this with or without your consent. So if you have been paid by someone else's insurance policy for an illness or injury the other person caused, your HMO has the right to recover from you the cost or value of any services the other person may have paid for or covered.

The rules for subrogation will be described in detail in your contract, but in general it works like this: If you receive a $25,000 settlement from another person's auto insurance company after an accident, and your HMO covered your emergency and follow-up care at a cost of $15,000, you will have to pay back to your HMO $15,000 out of your $25,000 settlement.

# 6

## Using a Point-of-Service Plan: When Non-Network Care Is a Covered Option

At this point, you should have a better understanding of how to get the most out of your HMO's care and coverage by following its "in-network" rules and procedures. As mentioned earlier, however, there is a variation on the standard HMO plan that might be available to you; it's called a "point-of-service" (POS) plan. POS plans combine the "in-network" rules of the standard HMO with "non-network" rules that give members the option to get care, on their own and without a referral, from doctors and other medical professionals outside their HMO's network (commonly called "non-network" or "non-participating" providers).

### IN-NETWORK CARE AND COVERAGE

In-network care and coverage rules for point-of-service plans are the same as for standard HMOs. You will be required to choose a primary care doctor from the plan's network, and your primary care doctor or your plan will provide, arrange, or authorize all of your care, except in life-threatening emergencies or when you travel. If you follow these rules, when you are inside or outside your plan's service area, your benefits will be covered at the highest level, usually with no deductibles, coinsurance or claim forms, and with relatively small copayments or visit fees for most of the care you receive (typically $5 to $15 for doctor visits and up to several hundred dollars for hospitalization).

## NON-NETWORK CARE AND COVERAGE

If you choose to get care from non-network providers, your coverage will look more like traditional fee-for-service health insurance. You will have to pay deductibles and coinsurance and you will have to file claim forms. Non-network care will cost you more than in-network care. In most point-of-service plans, non-network care and coverage work like this:

▶For the most part, your covered benefits—the kinds of medical care your plan will pay for—are the same as your in-network covered benefits. And the exclusions—what is not covered—are the same. This means that if your plan covers infertility services in network, it will cover them out of network. If it excludes cosmetic surgery in network because it is not "medically necessary," it will not pay for it out of network either. There is an important exception to this rule, however: Many point-of-service plans cover routine physical exams and preventive care like immunizations and inoculations *only* when you get them from an in-network HMO provider.

▶If you want to get care from a doctor or other medical professional who is outside your HMO's network, that is your choice. For instance, if you want to go to a particular non-network pediatrician, gynecologist, orthopedic surgeon, or cancer specialist, you can, without getting a referral or prior authorization.

►You can also go to a hospital of your own choice if you want to. You may want to choose a non-network hospital for its reputation, its convenience to your home, or because you are seeing a non-network specialist and it is the hospital to which he or she can admit patients.

►While you can make your own choice of hospitals, you will have to follow some non-network rules in order to be covered by your point-of-service plan. Typically, you will be required to notify your HMO prior to any nonemergency hospitalization. Also, your hospital admission will probably have to be "precertified." Precertification is the way your HMO determines whether your hospital admission, the services you will receive, and the length of your hospital stay are medically necessary and appropriate.

►These rules for notification and precertification apply for maternity care and for mental health and substance abuse care, as well as for other hospitalizations. Emergency hospital admissions will not have to be precertified, but you should make sure you notify your HMO soon after you are admitted.

►If you decide to get your medical care out of network, you will pay higher out-of-pocket costs in the form of deductibles and coinsurance. Your deductible means that your plan will not start paying for your care until you have paid a certain fixed amount each year, typically $200 to $500 per member or $400 to $1000 per family. Your coinsurance means that after the deductible amount is reached, your plan will pay a percent of the cost of your care and you will pay the rest. For instance, your plan might pay 75 percent and you pay 25 percent, or you might split the cost 80/20, or 60/40, after you meet the annual deductible. The higher your share is, the less expensive your POS plan premiums should be. Higher levels of cost sharing discourage members from choosing to get their care outside the HMO network, and in-network care is less expensive for you and the HMO.

▶There are dollar limits on the amount you will have to pay out of pocket for covered benefits each year. Once you have reached those limits, which are typically $2000 to $4000 a year, your plan will pay 100 percent of your non-network coverage. At the annual renewal date of your coverage, your deductible requirement and your out-of-pocket limits start all over again.

▶If your HMO requires precertification and you are hospitalized out of network without precertification, you will be responsible for even more of the cost of your care. Even if you follow the rules, of course, your personal costs for non-network deductibles and coinsurance are likely to be much higher than the copayments or visit fees you will pay if you stay in network.

▶You or your provider will have to file a claim in order to be paid back by your plan for non-network care. Claim forms are available through your employer. Be sure to keep records of all your deductible and coinsurance payments.

## OUT-OF-AREA COVERAGE FROM YOUR POS PLAN

What happens when you get out-of-area care can be a little confusing, because it is *always* provided outside of your HMO's network. Just remember that if you follow the in-network rules when you are out of area, you will be covered at the in-network level; if you don't, you will be covered at the non-network level. (Deductibles and coinsurance will apply.) Some examples:

►If you are pregnant and travel a few weeks before your due date, and you go into labor and deliver your baby in an out-of-area hospital, you will probably have to pay coinsurance at the non-network levels. Your HMO would say that your maternity hospitalization was care that could have been anticipated by you and provided in network by your HMO.

►If you are away from home and you decide to go to a famous cancer institute for tests, this would again be considered non-network care because you could have had the tests conducted by, or arranged and authorized by, your HMO.

►If you are in a car accident while traveling, your HMO will cover your hospitalization at the in-network level, because it is an emergency. However, if you choose to get your follow-up care from the out-of-area hospital or doctors, rather than having it provided by your HMO, you will get only non-network coverage.

## PREEXISTING-CONDITION LIMITATIONS

Some point-of-service plans have waiting periods or dollar limits for the coverage of preexisting medical conditions. If you or a member of your family has a disease, injury, or medical condition that was discovered or treated within a short period before your membership became effective, your plan might impose a waiting period before it will cover treatment of that condition, or cover it only up to a fixed dollar amount. These limitations might apply only to non-network care or to both in-network and non-network care.

## LIMITS ON BENEFIT PAYMENTS

There are two types of limitations your point-of-service plan may put on what it will pay for non-network care you receive. First of all, it will probably pay only "reasonable and customary" fees to any non-network doctor or hospital that takes care of you. For instance: Suppose a non-network doctor charges $500 for tests, but your POS plan decides that $400 is reasonable and customary. This means that if your POS plan pays 70 percent coinsurance after you pay your annual deductible, it will only reimburse the doctor for $280 instead of $350. If you're supposed to pay the difference, should you pay $150 or $220? Find out in advance what your plan's policy is and what your obligation will be.

Your plan may also limit the amount it will pay for covered benefits during each member's lifetime. For example, a plan may put a $100,000 limit on the amount it will pay for non-network care and a $1,000,000 limit on the total amount it will pay for all covered benefits. Although $100,000 may sound like a lot of money, there are many medical procedures that can cost that much. If you need an organ transplant, or bone marrow transplant, or very specialized heart surgery, and want to arrange for it yourself outside of your HMO's network, you could use up your entire lifetime non-network benefits with a single procedure or course of treatment.

## WHEN SHOULD YOU CHOOSE CARE OUTSIDE YOUR HMO's NETWORK?

Although point-of-service HMOs haven't been around for a long time, their experience so far is that members go out of network for only a very small percentage of their care; they get most of what they need in network. Still, members appreciate the flexibility that point-of-service plans offer, especially if they are used to traditional fee-for-service health insurance and they aren't ready to make the leap to a more restrictive (and less expensive) standard HMO, which offers only in-network benefits.

There are several reasons you might want to choose non-network care:

▶To stay with your own doctor: If you have had a long-time family doctor, a pediatrician who has cared for your children since birth, a gynecologist with whom you are very comfortable, or a specialist who has been treating you for years, it could be very hard to switch. If that favorite doctor is not part of your HMO's network of primary care doctors or referral specialists, you may be willing to pay more to continue the relationship, while using the HMO's network for the rest of your health care. Your POS plan should allow you to see your "old" doctor for some or all of the care you need. Remember, however, that you might still have to go to your HMO primary care doctor for routine preventive care unless you want to pay the entire cost yourself.

▶To get what you consider better quality of care: Another reason to go outside your HMO's network is that you think you can get better quality of care. Some doctors and some hospitals have reputations as the best in their communities for their specialties. If they are not part of your point-of-service plan's network, you still have the option of choosing them for your care. Since specialty and hospital care is very expensive, your out-of-pocket costs (coinsurance) could mount up quickly, so you should do some careful research before you make your decision.

▶To get care that is closer to home: If you or members of your family have to make frequent trips to the doctor, and your plan doesn't have in-network doctors close to your community, you may decide to establish a relationship with a local doctor who doesn't participate in your HMO and is therefore non-network.

▶To get better access and service: If you are frustrated by your ability to get an appointment with a specialist who is part of your HMO's network, or you think you are not being listened to, taken seriously enough, or treated with courtesy and respect, you have the option to make your own arrangements for care. You can also go outside the plan's network for a second opinion from a doctor of your choice.

---

### Before You Go Out of Network . . .

As you think about going out of network for care, there are several important points to keep in mind.

- Make sure you understand all of what your HMO's network has to offer; there may be excellent in-network specialists or hospitals that can meet your needs if you can get referred to them.
- Be clear in your own mind about how you are judging the quality of the non-network doctor or hospital you choose. Is your decision based on what is really important to you?
- Make sure the course of treatment your non-network doctor recommends is covered by your plan's benefits.
- If it is covered, ask in advance how much you are likely to pay for out-of-pocket coinsurance costs, not just for the first appointment but for your entire course of treatment.
- Make sure you follow your plan's rules regarding non-network referrals, authorization, or hospital precertification and the filing of claims.

---

# DON'T LET YOUR CARE BECOME UNCOORDINATED

One of the reasons HMOs want you to choose a primary care doctor and have that doctor provide or arrange all of your nonemergency care is so that your care will be well-coordinated. This means there should be excellent, ongoing communication about your medical care among your primary care doctor, any specialists you see, and any other medical professionals who take care of you. Good communication can help ensure that you get appropriate care in a timely fashion; that you are well informed about your overall course of treatment; that no aspect of your care falls through the cracks; that services or tests are not repeated unnecessarily; and that follow-up care is well planned. Some HMOs have medical records systems that make your medical history easily available to anyone who provides you with medical care. When you decide to get care out of network, these important lines of communication and coordination can be broken.

If you want your care to be well coordinated, you will have to take responsibility for letting your primary care doctor know when you are getting non-network care, and why. You should also make sure that reports or medical records for care you receive out of network are sent to your primary care doctor. Ask your HMO doctor, your non-network doctor, or your HMO's member service department how they can help make sure your care is well coordinated.

CASE EXAMPLE:
IS IT TIME TO GO OUT OF NETWORK?

*Roy had a problem with severe back pain that was keeping him from carrying on his normal activities, like biking and gardening. His HMO primary care doctor referred Roy to an orthopedic specialist, who examined him and recommended some exercises he could use to reduce his pain. After a few weeks, it became apparent that his self-treatment just wasn't working, and after a second visit to the specialist, he felt he was still not making progress.*

*A friend at work told Roy that she had an orthopedic specialist she had been seeing for years, and she was sure he could get an appointment within a week. She said her doctor would probably arrange for a high-tech MRI scan to pinpoint Roy's problem and would be more willing to operate than the HMO specialist. Roy was frustrated and in pain, and with his point-of-service plan he could go to this non-network doctor and still be covered for 70 percent of the cost. What should he do?*

*Since Roy would have to pay more for non-network care, his first step should have been to make sure he had done what he could to get the care he needed in network. He decided to talk to his primary care doctor about his frustrations and concerns and make it clear that he was considering non-network care if he couldn't get some relief. He asked his doctor to get directly involved in helping with his specialty care.*

*Within a week, Roy's primary care doctor had made a second referral, this time to a pain clinic at a local hospital that was part of his HMO's network. To his surprise, he discovered that his friend's orthopedic specialist practiced at the pain clinic, and that, rather than recommend surgery or an MRI, the doctor decided to try a cortisone shot. This time, Roy got immediate relief, and two months later, the pain hadn't returned.*

# 7

## Making Your HMO Work for Your Good Health: Sixteen Areas of Special Concern

Changing your health care plan can be a source of great anxiety if you are being treated for a serious illness; becoming seriously ill can be much more traumatic if you are unsure how to get the best care from your HMO. In this chapter, you'll find out how to handle both situations: what to do if you join an HMO in the middle of a serious illness, and how to get good care for a serious illness that is diagnosed after you join. You'll also find information on some types of health care—like maternity and pediatric care—that are more routine, but that require an especially clear and thorough understanding of the care and coverage your HMO provides.

None of the information in this chapter is meant to be medical advice; you should always consult with a medical professional about any medical concerns you have. What you'll find here are tips on the questions you should ask and the issues you should discuss with your doctor and other clinicians who might take care of you. These guidelines assume that you choose, or are referred to, a clinician who participates in your HMO's network. However, if you are a member of a point-of-service plan and you choose to get non-network care for your condition, you can still use the information in this chapter to help you get the best possible care.

If you have a serious illness when you join an HMO and you have to switch primary care doctors or specialists, ask the HMO whether they have a clinical transition program to help ensure that you get high-quality uninterrupted care for your condition. (See also "What If You Are Pregnant or Being Treated for a Serious Illness," starting on page 66).

## ADOLESCENT CARE

Today's adolescents are at risk. Sexually transmitted diseases, eating disorders, drug and alcohol abuse, stress, depression, sexual abuse, violence, sports injuries—all afflict American teenagers at what seems to be a frightening rate. Whether these problems are really on the rise, or only more out in the open, health care professionals are paying much greater attention to the special needs of adolescents.

Caring for adolescents typically requires more than simply taking care of their physical health. Adolescents and teenagers experience a host of emotional ups and downs along with physical changes. A primary care doctor who cares for adolescents (usually a pediatrician or family practitioner) and who understands their emotions can be a great resource for the whole family, and can help you and your child safely navigate an often stormy period.

When does a child become an adolescent? For many parents, the answer seems instinctive and obvious: You know one when you see one. ("Help! My kid is starting to act like an adolescent!") But in today's society, the problems we have listed above seem to be affecting many children at a younger and younger age. Since health care plays only one small (but very important) part in a child's development, it is up to the parents, or parent, and, if possible, the child, to decide when adolescent issues should be a matter of concern. Your personal beliefs and values, and your home, school, and community environments will all play a role.

As your child approaches adulthood, she has a right to confidential treatment from her doctor. Many parents find it hard not knowing what their child might be discussing with the doctor. But finding a doctor you trust, and allowing your child to develop an open and honest relationship with that doctor, are among the best ways to assure that your child will seek and receive care when it's needed.

### Questions That Can Help You Choose a Doctor for Your Adolescent Child

◆ Are there adolescent specialists, or other doctors with a strong interest in this age group available in your HMO's network?

◆ Does your HMO have a teen clinic? Are there health education classes or materials for your child and for you?

◆ Are there doctors whose office environments are most suitable for teens?

◆ Is there easy access for a child who may need counseling or other mental health services?

### Things to Discuss with Your Adolescent's HMO Clinician

◆ Whether there are standard topics the doctor discusses with adolescent patients during office visits; whether the doctor follows a set of treatment guidelines, such as the American Medical Association's *Guidelines for Adolescent Preventive Services,* published in 1993.

◆ What the parents' role will be in the relationship between the doctor and the child.

◆ How the doctor balances her obligation to protect the child's privacy with the parents' wish to be involved in the child's care.

◆ Your feelings about difficult teenage issues like sexuality and birth control, abortion, homosexuality, smoking, and drug or alcohol use. You may want to ask the doctor what she would do if your child came to her with one of these problems.

◆ Whether your child can get an appointment on her own, and whether someone will make sure she understands how the HMO works if she needs additional care and wants to pursue it on her own; also what might happen if she can't afford the copayment.

◆ Any special services or educational programs that are available for teens, like courses on pregnancy prevention, AIDS awareness, or drug and alcohol use.

◆ What kind of individual or family counseling is available should the need arise.

◆ Whether your HMO offers programs or courses to help you support and communicate with your adolescent.

◆ Whether the doctor or the HMO can help link your adolescent with social services or peer-group programs outside the HMO network.

## AIDS

People with AIDS are living twice as long today as they were ten years ago, thanks to new treatments, new medications, and new understanding of the disease. Naturally, HMO members who are HIV positive or who have AIDS want to know that health care services that can extend the length and the quality of their lives will be available to them.

If you want to be tested for the HIV virus, speak with your HMO primary care physician. He or she can make the arrangements you need, and should be able to reassure you about confidentiality surrounding the test itself and the results.

If you have already been tested and know you are HIV positive or have AIDS, your need for medical care depends on how far your disease has progressed. You may require relatively minor medical treatment, or you may be in need of a broad range of services. Most health care for people living with HIV focuses on trying to prevent or treat AIDS-related illnesses, and on keeping people as active as possible. Since AIDS-related diseases take many different forms, their treatment may require several types of specialists, including infectious disease specialists, oncologists, pulmonologists, dermatologists, and ophthalmologists. When you join an HMO, you'll want to be sure the doctors, hospitals, and other providers in the HMO network are experienced and equipped to give you the care and services you may need, ranging from counseling to treatment to home care.

Your primary care physician will provide or authorize most of your care for HIV and AIDS; he or she may refer you to specialists for some of your care, but will most likely remain responsible for coordinating the care provided by any other clinicians you see. Your relationship with your primary care physician, and with the specialists to whom you are referred, will be an important part of how you feel about the care you receive.

If you are under the care of a doctor when you join the HMO, check with him to see if he is part of the HMO's primary care network, or might be able to join. If he isn't, you will need to choose a doctor who is affiliated with the HMO. If you find out that you are HIV positive after you are already an HMO member, remember that you have the option of changing primary care doctors to make sure you have one who can best meet your needs.

## Questions That Can Help You Choose Your Doctor

- ◆ Which primary care physicians have the most experience with HIV and AIDS?
- ◆ If you are referred to a specialist, what role will your primary care physician continue to play in your care?
- ◆ Are there other members of the doctor's clinical team (nurses, nurse practitioners, physicians' assistants) who will be involved in your care? Who is available to see you when your doctor isn't?
- ◆ What kind of AIDS education programs and clinical protocols are the HMO's doctors involved in?
- ◆ What hospitals are used and how are admissions arranged? If you have a preference, you may be able to choose an HMO doctor who admits there.

## Things to Discuss with Your HMO Clinician

- ◆ His approach to the management of AIDS—and yours—including treatment options, how you will be informed of new treatments, where you prefer to be treated, and how your doctor can coordinate his care with any AIDS-related services you might be receiving outside your HMO.
- ◆ His or the HMO's policy about experimental treatments, and how you would get access to clinical trials.

◆ Any religious, cultural, or philosophical beliefs you have that may impact the kind of care you want.

◆ Whether your HMO has a centralized AIDS treatment program that coordinates services for AIDS patients and that employs clinicians with special expertise and experience in AIDS.

◆ The kinds of counseling, social services, support groups, or educational programs that are available from your HMO for yourself, members of your family, or your partner.

◆ How confidentiality is handled; any separate ways in which the HMO assures that a patient's HIV status is protected information; in how many places this information resides.

◆ What you should do in an emergency, especially at night or on weekends; who is available when your doctor isn't.

◆ Home care or hospice care that is available through your HMO and what is covered.

◆ How you could create advance directives, such as a living will or health care proxy, if you want to plan for when you might be too sick to make decisions on your own behalf.

## ASTHMA

Asthma is a chronic respiratory disease that often causes coughing, wheezing, and/or shortness of breath. It may lead to sudden acute episodes when breathing becomes very difficult. Too often undertreated, asthma is the leading cause of hospitalization and emergency room care for children and of time lost from school and work for children and adults. It is estimated that childhood asthma causes more than 10 million missed days of school and 200,000 hospitalizations a year in the United States, many of which could be avoided.

Asthma cannot be cured, but experts agree that careful and appropriate management can greatly lessen its impact. People with asthma can use medicine to relieve their symptoms, and they can learn how to manage episodes that might lead to emergency hospitalization. With proper care, they can lead normal lives.

If you or your child has asthma, you should choose a primary care doctor within the HMO who is knowledgeable about the newest and best ways to manage asthma. If you are under a doctor's care for asthma when you join an HMO, find out if you can continue to see him, either as your primary care doctor or by referral for specialty care. If you have to change doctors, or if you or your child is diagnosed with asthma after you are already an HMO member, you will want to make sure you have a primary care doctor who can provide you with the best care.

Depending on the severity of your asthma (or your child's), your primary care doctor may involve other specialists in your care. He may consult or refer you to an allergist, a pulmonologist, or a team of physician and nurse specialists, but he should remain responsible for coordinating your specialty care and for helping you with the everyday management of your condition.

*Questions That Can Help You Choose a Primary Care Doctor, for Yourself or Your Child*

- ◆ Which HMO doctors are the most knowledgeable and experienced in treating children or adults with asthma?
- ◆ How is the practice organized? What other clinicians might you or your child see? Who covers for your doctor

when he is away? How can you meet the other clinicians in the practice?

◆ What specialists are used and how are referrals made?

◆ What hospitals are used and how are admissions arranged? If you have a preference, you may be able to choose a doctor who admits there.

◆ What happens in an emergency? Who is available at nights or on weekends?

## Things to Discuss with Your HMO Clinicians

◆ Their approach to the management of asthma; the recommended strategy for preventing serious attacks, emergency room visits, or hospitalizations; whether specialists will be involved in your care, and how.

◆ Any questions or concerns you may have about medicines that are being prescribed or recommended for asthma management or treatment.

◆ Any medications you or your child may already be taking.

◆ The role parents and other family members can play in helping a child manage asthma.

◆ Any publications or other educational materials that can help you understand asthma and how it can be managed.

◆ The kinds of training, support, and equipment that are available to help assess and manage your condition or your child's condition (like peak flow meters).

◆ The impact of the home environment; any factors that might aggravate asthmatic symptoms.

◆ If there are smokers in the home (which aggravates asthma), whether there are classes to help them quit smoking.

◆ What you should do in an emergency; how you will know when you have to call your HMO or doctor before getting help and when you should get immediate help, by calling 911 or going to a hospital emergency room.

◆ What will happen if you or your child needs to be hospitalized; the role your primary care doctor will play during hospitalization.

◆ Any religious, cultural, philosophical, or family issues that will impact the kind of care you want for yourself or your child.

# CANCER

Few things are more frightening than hearing that you or someone you love has cancer. Finding a doctor or doctors in whom you have confidence will help alleviate some of your fear.

Cancer occurs in many different forms, and it can affect many different organs and parts of the body. There are also many different treatment options, including minor or major surgery, chemotherapy, and radiation therapy. It is almost certain, therefore, that your primary care physician will refer you to one or more specialists, including an oncologist, surgeon, or radiologist, for your cancer treatment.

Excellent communication and coordination are essential in the diagnosis and treatment of cancer. If you feel there has not been swift and thorough follow-up after your diagnosis, that your HMO or your doctor is moving too slowly, that you are not getting straight answers, that you are not being listened to, or that your doctor is not plugged in to the best treatment options, your frustration, anger, and fear will be multiplied. You, your primary care doctor, and any specialists you see should ideally feel like a team working together toward your good health. Your relationship should be strong and comfortable, and you should feel encouraged to participate as much as possible in decisions about your care. You and members of your family may also need special support to get through the psychological and physical burdens cancer treatment can produce.

If you are already in the midst of a treatment plan for cancer when you join an HMO, find out whether your doctor is in the HMO network, or if the HMO would let you continue seeing her until your treatment is finished. If not, you will have to choose a doctor in the HMO network in order to have your care covered. If that is the case, find out if your HMO has a clinical transition program to ensure that you get high-quality, uninterrupted treatment.

While you will probably have other medical needs as well, your cancer is likely to dominate your life for some period of time. So if you are diagnosed with cancer after you become an HMO member, you will want to make certain that your primary care doctor is familiar with your kind of cancer and has the kind of communications skills you require. This may require changing your primary care doctor.

## Questions That Can Help You Choose a Doctor

- ◆ Which primary care physicians have the most experience caring for patients with your kind of cancer, and access to the most current treatment protocols?
- ◆ What role will your primary care doctor play in treating your cancer? What roles do specialists play?

◆ What roles do other clinicians (nurses, nurse practitioners, physicians' assistants) play in cancer treatment? Who is available to see you when your doctor isn't?

◆ What hospitals are used for treatment of your kind of cancer? For surgery only, or for chemotherapy and radiation therapy too? If you have a preference, you may be able to choose a doctor who admits there.

## Things to Discuss with Your HMO Clinician

◆ What kind of clinical research or national treatment protocols your doctor has access to.

◆ Her approach, and yours, to the treatment and management of your kind of cancer.

◆ How referrals work; how to be sure your care is covered.

◆ How referral decisions are made; to whom she is likely to refer you and why.

◆ If you will be referred to an oncologist, which oncologists are most experienced with your kind of cancer, and what their credentials are.

◆ Who will be responsible for overseeing your treatment plan, and for communicating each step or decision with you and with other clinicians on your "team." How that communication among clinicians takes place, and what your role should be in facilitating it.

◆ The kind of involvement you want in decisions about your care.

◆ How your family will be involved and supported.

◆ The kinds of counseling, social services, or educational programs that are available.

- How to get second opinions about your diagnosis or treatment.
- Any alternative therapies that you are interested in learning about or trying.
- Your preferences about pain management.
- What you should do in an emergency, especially at night or on weekends; who is available when your doctor isn't.
- What kind of home care or hospice care is available through your HMO, and what is covered.
- Whether or not you have or want to create a living will, advance directives, or health care proxy in case you become too sick to make decisions on your own behalf.

## CHRONIC OR PROLONGED ILLNESS

Many long-term chronic illnesses, especially infectious or inflammatory diseases like Lyme disease, Crohn's disease, or chronic fatigue syndrome, have several troublesome characteristics in common. The cause is often unclear; the symptoms are vague and varied, making diagnosis long and difficult; treatments to relieve the symptoms sometimes work and sometimes don't, with their success varying from patient to patient or even for the same patient over time; and, while the symptoms can weaken or disappear for months or even years at a time, the illness may never really go away.

Many other chronic disorders have clearer origins and treatment options, but still require lifelong management. This description applies to a wide range of conditions, including lupus, colitis, glaucoma, endometriosis, multiple sclerosis, eczema, chronic back pain, allergies, respiratory diseases, and a host of other disorders. The common thread in this list is that these are ailments with which patients must learn to live.

The permanence of these illnesses, and the shortage of clear answers surrounding their causes and treatments, are the ideal breeding ground for frustration, anger, and fear for patients and their families. More than most illnesses, chronic disorders require a strong working partnership between doctor and patient. Your role in the partnership is to provide information to your doctor. Owing to the vague and variable nature of some of these disorders, what you tell your doctor about your symptoms and your response to treatments will be crucial to his ability to help you manage your illness; the more detailed information you provide, the better. (Many patients with chronic disorders keep a detailed journal of symptoms, medications, treatments, and reactions for this very reason.) Your doctor's role in the partnership is to listen to you, to understand your symptoms and your concerns, and to include you in the decision-making process. Anything less than an equal partnership will probably result in frustration for you both.

Your HMO primary care physician will "own" your care: he will provide it directly, or coordinate with specialists, who will provide it as needed. If you have a disorder that requires the care of several specialists, then the role that your primary care doctor plays is essential to making sure your care is not fragmented. While each specialist may have a thorough understanding of a specific aspect of your illness, your primary care doctor will see "the big picture": how your care is integrated across specialties. This is a particular strength of HMOs versus so-called "fee-for-service" medicine.

If you have a chronic disorder and are joining an HMO, you may want to choose a primary care doctor who has experience and expertise with your illness. If you are already an HMO member and are diagnosed with a chronic disorder, you will probably want to stay with your existing primary care doctor, who knows you and your health history. Of course you should be able to change primary care physicians any time you wish.

## Questions That Can Help You Choose Your Doctor

◆ Who has the most experience with your particular disorder?

◆ If you are referred to specialists, who might they be? And what role will your primary care physician play?

◆ Does this doctor practice in a team with other clinicians? Who else might be involved in providing your care? Who is available when the doctor isn't?

◆ What hospitals are used? If you have a preference, you may be able to choose a doctor who admits there.

## Things to Discuss with Your HMO Clinician

◆ His approach to managing your illness, and his experience with various treatments, either traditional or alternative.

◆ Your experiences with your illness and treatments; your preferences if you have any.

◆ How your relationship will work best for both of you; how decisions will be made.

◆ Educational materials or support groups that are available for you and/or your family.

◆ What you should do in an emergency.

◆ How to plan ahead should your illness become more severe or disabling.

# DIABETES

Diabetes, a disorder in which food is not properly converted into energy for the body, is a complex disease that, in some patients, affects nearly every organ of the body. Estimated to occur in about six million Americans, diabetes comes in two forms. Type I, or insulin-dependent diabetes, requires lifelong treatment with insulin, as well as careful attention to diet and exercise. This type of diabetes is often hereditary, and is usually first diagnosed during childhood or adolescence. Type II, the more common form of diabetes, generally occurs first in adulthood, and can usually be controlled through appropriate diet and exercise.

Medical experts today advise that diabetes of either type should be more aggressively managed than it has been in years past. This often means more frequent monitoring of blood sugar, closer attention to diet and exercise, and, for patients with insulin-dependent diabetes, more frequent use of insulin in smaller doses. Many diabetics have reacted positively to being more directly involved in the management of their disease. Although this may take a great deal more effort on their part, it does not interfere with their ability to lead a normal life, and in many instances their feelings about their quality of life improves when their diabetes is under better control.

If you have diabetes, you are more involved in monitoring, treating, and managing your disease than patients with many other disorders. You are the key to your own continuing good health, because you must be constantly vigilant about any symptoms suggesting that your glucose level is too high or too low. For this reason, it is essential that you and your doctor form a partnership in the management of your health. If you are already under treatment for diabetes when you join an HMO, you should check to see if your current doctor is part of the HMO network. If so, you won't have to choose a new doctor. If not, you will need to choose a doctor who is in the HMO network.

In some cases, diabetic care is provided by a primary care physician; in others, an endocrinologist or other specialist may be involved. If you do see a specialist, you will need to be referred by your primary care physician in order to be covered. You should be sure you understand your benefits, in particular, how to get a referral and whether you will need to get your referral renewed from time to time, and which medications, supplies, or devices are covered.

Whether you are diagnosed with diabetes before or after you join an HMO, you will want to make sure you feel comfortable and confident that your primary care physician can treat and manage your condition, and can give you access to the specialists you need.

## Questions That Can Help You Choose Your Doctor

◆ Who will provide your care as it relates to diabetes? Your primary care physician? A specialist?

◆ Which of the HMO's primary care physicians are most experienced and knowledgeable about diabetes?

◆ If you have special needs (if you are pregnant, trying to get pregnant, or if the patient is a child), which doctors are most experienced with these types of patients?

◆ If you see a specialist, what role will your primary care physician continue to play in your care?

◆ What roles do other clinicians (nurses, nurse practitioners, physicians' assistants) play? Who is available to see you when your doctor isn't?

◆ What hospitals are used for the treatment of diabetes? If you have a preference, you may be able to choose a doctor who admits there.

*Things to Discuss with Your HMO Clinician*

◆ His or her approach to the management of diabetes; whether your HMO has centralized services for diabetes care.

◆ What the relationship will be among your primary care provider, specialists, and you.

◆ Whether formal protocols or standards of diabetes care have been adopted by your HMO or your doctor.

◆ Educational materials that are available to help you manage your diabetes; whether nutrition or exercise counseling are available.

◆ Whether there is a formal reminder system for regular vision, dental, or other exams that are important for diabetics.

◆ What you should do in an emergency, especially at night or on weekends.

◆ Any clinical trials or research projects that your doctor may have access to.

# DISABILITIES

Millions of Americans have disabilities of one kind or another. Some are visible (like amputations, blindness, a tracheotomy), others are not (like learning disabilities or severe agoraphobia). Some patients are able to work, play, and live a fairly normal life with their disabilities; others are much more restricted in their activities. Some conditions improve with time, while others get worse.

Common to all long-term disabilities is the need for careful medical, psychological, and financial management. You and your family will require ongoing support, information, and guidance, as well as medical interventions and treatments.

All HMOs share a goal to keep their members healthy through aggressive preventive care. This is more than good medicine; because the care HMO members receive is prepaid, the HMO is collecting the same premium from healthy people and from people in need of extensive and expensive care. Healthy patients help the HMO save money; patients with long-term disabilities generally do not, and for this reason these patients can often end up feeling that the HMO doesn't really want them as members.

This is all the more reason why it's important to find a physician in the HMO who will provide you with ongoing care, support, and empathy in an unequivocally positive way. Because your disability may require lifelong care, it's also important that you try to establish a long-term relationship with your primary care doctor.

Depending on the nature and severity of your disability, you may also need additional supports, like medical equipment, supplies, or care at home, technological devices to help you communicate (computers, TTY machines), or a special vehicle in which to travel. While most of these things will not be covered by your HMO, you should be able to get some guidance and assistance in identifying your needs and finding a source for purchasing special items, as well as organizations that might help you pay for them if you cannot afford them yourself.

As an HMO member, your primary care doctor will be chiefly responsible for your care. What care he doesn't provide himself he will coordinate, referring you to appropriate specialists, conferring with them, and managing the overall provision of your care. If you are new to the HMO, you should try to choose a doctor with whom you will be comfortable over the long haul. If you become disabled while you are already an HMO member, your current primary care doctor may be best prepared to care for you, since he already knows you. Either way, you need to feel comfortable and confident about your doctor. If you don't, choose a different doctor, one who inspires you to feel that way.

## Questions That Can Help You Choose Your Doctor

- ◆ Who has the most experience with your particular disability?
- ◆ If you are referred to specialists, who might they be? And what role will your primary care physician play?
- ◆ Does this doctor practice in a team with other clinicians? Who else might be involved in providing your care? Who is available when the doctor isn't?
- ◆ If you are housebound, how will you receive your care?
- ◆ What hospitals are used? If you have a preference, you may be able to choose a doctor who admits there.
- ◆ In what other settings might you receive care? Rehabilitation hospitals? Skilled nursing facilities?

## Things to Discuss with Your HMO Clinician

- ◆ His or her approach to managing your disability.
- ◆ Your experiences with your disability, your fears, your hopes, your preferences.
- ◆ How your relationship will work best for both of you; how decisions will be made.
- ◆ How your care will be coordinated among specialists, or in different settings such as your physician's office, a hospital, or a skilled nursing facility.

◆ The kinds of equipment or special devices that are covered, and how decisions will be made about what your needs are.

◆ Under what circumstances home care is covered.

◆ Educational materials or support groups that are available for you and/or your family.

◆ What you should do in an emergency.

◆ How to plan ahead should your disability become more severe or your abilities more limited.

◆ What kind of long-term care is covered, and what the alternatives are when and if coverage ends.

◆ Sources of support, either psychological or financial, in the HMO or in the community.

## HEART DISEASE

Studies show that Americans are eating less fat than they were ten years ago, and there has been a significant drop in the average American's blood cholesterol level. That's the good news. The bad news is that coronary artery disease is still the leading cause of death in our nation.

Coronary artery disease, in which plaque builds up on the walls of the arteries, decreasing the flow of blood and oxygen to the heart, is the most common form of heart disease. It is also often preventable, through proper diet, blood pressure control, exercise, and healthy habits (like reducing stress or managing it better, and not smoking).

Chest pain is the most common symptom of heart disease, and people often confuse it with other chest pains, like heartburn or pleurisy. Whenever you feel chest pain, whether you imagine you are a candidate for heart disease or not, you should err on the side of caution: seek medical help or advice.

Your HMO has rules about what to do if you need urgent care (usually defined as care within twenty-four to forty-eight hours), and what to do if you need emergency, or immediate, care. Sometimes it is hard to distinguish which is which, but most HMOs regard chest pain as an emergency, in which members can seek immediate care without calling first for authorization. Whatever your HMO's policy, you or someone with you should call your HMO doctor if you are seen in a hospital emergency room for chest pain so he or she can manage any care you may require.

If you have already been diagnosed or treated for a heart condition when you join an HMO, you'll probably find that your primary care doctor will assume more direct responsibility for your care, working collaboratively with a cardiac specialist. If you've had bypass surgery or angioplasty, for instance, your primary relationship may have been with a cardiologist. But because the HMO philosophy of care is built around the relationship between a patient and a primary care physician, he or she will most likely be responsible for providing or coordinating all your care, including your cardiac care.

If your needs are not complex, your primary care doctor should be able to provide all or most of the cardiac care you need. This shouldn't mean you will be getting less expert care: many types of cardiac care are best provided by an internist or family practitioner. (You might even be able to choose a primary care doctor with subspecialty training in cardiology.) In addition, your primary care physician knows you best, and has the broadest view of all the physical and emotional issues that affect your health.

However, your primary care physician should refer you to a cardiologist when necessary, and should continue to oversee and coordinate your care. If these relationships are well managed, and if communication between the two doctors and with you is good, then you will have the best of both worlds.

## Questions That Can Help You Choose Your Doctor

◆ Which HMO primary care doctors are most experienced in treating your kind of condition?

◆ Which primary care doctors have access to one or more board certified cardiologists who have experience with your kind of condition?

◆ What role will the cardiologist play in caring for you? How will your primary and specialty care be coordinated?

◆ What hospitals do the HMO's cardilogists use? If you have a preference, you may want to choose a primary care doctor who can refer you to a cardiologist who admits there.

◆ If you wish to pursue less traditional treatments, like meditation or vitamin therapy, which doctor is likely to be most supportive?

## Things to Discuss with Your HMO Clinician

◆ What treatment options are available, and the benefits and risks of each.

◆ How decisions are made to do certain procedures (like catheterization, angioplasty, bypass surgery, insertion of a pacemaker).

◆ How you can get a second opinion (and have it covered by the HMO).

◆ Any interest you may have in less traditional treatments like meditation or vitamin therapy.

◆ What you should do in an emergency, especially at night or on weekends; how the HMO defines urgent versus emergency care for coverage purposes.

- Who is available when your cardiologist isn't.
- If you are a heart transplant candidate, how the waiting list is managed.
- From whom you will get follow-up care after a cardiac procedure (the cardiologist or your primary care physician).
- What kind of follow-up care you will need, what regular appointments you should anticipate.

## FAMILY PLANNING AND INFERTILITY

The scope and definition of family planning have changed dramatically in recent years. Family planning includes medical services that help a woman achieve or avoid pregnancy and childbirth. New technologies for genetic testing, for the treatment of infertility, and for birth control and abortion have made this an increasingly complex area, both medically and ethically.

What your HMO covers in this area may be determined in large part by your employer or by state law. For instance, some employers exclude abortion or birth control coverage for their employees and some states require coverage of in vitro fertilization (IVF) and similar infertility treatments, while others do not. But beyond what is included or excluded in your member contract may be a lot of very difficult questions and gray areas that you will have to explore if you want to get the most out of your HMO for family planning and infertility services.

Family planning services that are typically covered when they are provided or authorized by your HMO doctor or HMO include routine examinations, laboratory tests, pregnancy testing, infertility counseling and some types of infertility treatment, genetic counseling and some types of genetic testing, birth control counseling and some types of birth control, voluntary sterilization (but not reversal of voluntary sterilization), and abortion.

The phrase "and some types of . . ." is your clue that benefits may differ from plan to plan or state to state or that you may find that your HMO has guidelines that define how extensive your coverage will be. If these services include the use of prescription drugs, the extent of your coverage may also depend on whether or not you have your HMO's prescription drug benefit.

Since family planning is such a personal and emotionally trying aspect of your health care, you should make sure you understand what your options are, how they will be covered, and how to gain access to them.

## More on Infertility

Couples who have been diagnosed with infertility (generally defined as the inability to conceive a child normally in a year's time) are often able to reach their goal with the help of medical intervention. Sometimes there is a simple problem requiring a simple solution, and the treatment is easy, fast, and successful. Other times, diagnosis of the problem can take months or even years; treatment can be lengthy and varied. Sometimes the diagnosis is "unexplained infertility."

If you and your partner feel you are in need of infertility diagnosis or treatment, check with your primary care or ob/gyn doctor. He or she may be able to diagnose your problem simply and quickly. If you need more involved care and treatment, you may be referred to an infertility specialist.

If you are already involved in infertility tests or treatment when you join an HMO, you will have to choose a doctor in the HMO network in order for your care to be covered fully. (If you are a member of a point-of-service plan, you can choose to receive covered infertility care outside the HMO network and pay higher out-of-pocket costs.) Check to see if the doctor you have been seeing is in the HMO's network, or if the HMO will allow you to continue seeing your doctor until your treatment is complete. Chances are the answer will be no, so you will need to choose an HMO doctor in whom you will feel confident. The primary care doctor you choose will either provide the care you receive or refer you to an infertility specialist for your care.

Be sure to check with your HMO to find out what is covered. Even if your HMO covers infertility treatment, you may not be covered if you are not married, if you are beyond a specified age, or if both partners are not HMO members. Make sure you understand your benefits.

## Questions That Can Help You Choose Your Doctor

◆ What role does your primary care doctor play in diagnosing and treating your infertility? What role does a specialist play?

◆ Which primary care doctors have the most experience caring for infertile couples?

◆ Is it important for you and your partner to choose the same doctor?

◆ Where will you go for treatment? Will you be referred to another doctor, and if so, will your primary care doctor stay involved with your treatment?

◆ Does the HMO track its pregnancy success rates? If so, which specialist has the best record for successful pregnancies and births? Can you be referred to him or her?

## Things to Discuss with Your HMO Clinician

- Any infertility benefits limitations or exclusions imposed by your HMO contract; how they will affect your course of treatment.
- Who will be responsible for your overall care as it relates to infertility; who will be available to answer your questions.
- What is involved in diagnosing your infertility (sometimes called a "fertility workup").
- The kinds of treatment options that are available; their success rates; how decisions will be made about which treatments you will receive; and what will be the likely schedule for your treatment(s).
- At what age your coverage or treatment might be ended.
- How many attempts at conception the HMO will cover, and how "attempt" is defined.
- How often you will be allowed to receive treatment (every cycle, or every other).
- Ethical and philosophical issues around the use of donor sperm or eggs.
- Safeguards against disease in donor sperm or eggs.
- How you can get a second opinion.
- What happens if you have eggs or embryos left over after your treatment.
- The odds of having multiples (twins, triplets, or more).
- Any philosophical, religious, or cultural beliefs you have that may affect the kind of care you wish to receive.
- What support groups or counseling resources are available to help you cope with the stress of infertility and its treatment.

◆ Written or other educational materials that are available from your doctor or your HMO.

◆ What ongoing arrangements will be made for your care if you become pregnant.

## MATERNITY CARE

One of the most attractive features of HMOs has always been their comprehensive coverage of prenatal care and childbirth. The fact that a woman can have frequent visits to her doctor and all the necessary tests after becoming pregnant, take advantage of childbirth, breast-feeding, and newborn care education classes, have her child delivered and receive follow-up and nursery care, and then bring her infant in for well-baby care and vaccinations—all with virtually no out-of-pocket expenses—has amazed and delighted people who were used to the cost and restrictions of traditional health insurance. Still, there are many things a pregnant woman should do to take full advantage of the care and coverage HMOs offer.

Your prenatal care can begin as soon as it is confirmed that you are pregnant. You should talk to, or schedule an appointment with, your HMO primary care doctor or other clinician to begin planning for the months ahead. If your HMO has offered you an obstetrician/gynecologist as a primary care doctor, he or she will probably follow your care throughout your pregnancy and, if possible, your delivery. If not, your primary care clinician may provide some of your early prenatal care before referring you to an obstetrician or midwife.

If you are already pregnant and under the care of an obstetrician or midwife when you join an HMO, you may be reluctant to find a new one. Fortunately, most pregnancies are uncomplicated, and changing caregivers during the course of a pregnancy generally does not present any unusual medical challenges.

While most HMOs will not let you continue seeing your previous provider if she is not affiliated with the HMO, you should ask if that is possible, especially if you are in the later stages of pregnancy or if you have other health factors that put you at higher risk for complications. If you can't continue seeing your previous obstetrician or midwife, your HMO primary care doctor should be able to help you find one within the HMO's network with whom you can establish a good relationship. As with any medical condition, it's important that your obstetrical provider know as much of your medical history as possible. You should make sure that all of your medical records relating to this pregnancy, prior pregnancies, and any other care that might affect your pregnancy are transferred to your new clinician.

You may want to base your choice simply on which provider has the most time available to see patients. But if you have some specific preferences (a female, a doctor with a particular type of experience or philosophy, a midwife), you should try to find out who best meets your criteria.

Your primary care doctor, obstetrician, or midwife will probably have admitting privileges at a single maternity hospital, and that is where you will be scheduled to deliver. If your HMO has more than one maternity hospital in its network, and you have a strong preference for a particular one—for instance, one you've used before or one that has birthing or visiting policies you like—you will need to make sure the clinician you choose has admitting privileges there.

At some point in your pregnancy, you will be asked to choose a primary care doctor (a pediatrician or family practitioner) for your newborn. If possible, you should discuss arrangements for newborn care with your obstetrician or midwife and your child's pediatrician before you deliver. And don't forget to enroll your newborn in your HMO. You will probably have to notify your HMO (the member service department) no more than thirty days after your child's birth.

Now, a word about postpartum care (care after the birth of your child). When you were born, your mother probably stayed in the hospital a full week or more and brought you home to the waiting arms of a grandmother or other family member, who pampered you and your mother for a few more weeks until she "got on her feet." Times have changed, and hospital stays of twenty-four to forty-eight hours following an uncomplicated vaginal delivery have become the norm (and three to four days for a cesarean delivery). Many women prefer to return to the comfort and relative peace of their own homes as soon as possible, so they and their families can begin to get to know the new baby. Many HMOs provide some kind of follow-up care and instructions during those first few days at home to make sure the new mother and baby are doing well. Check with your HMO to find out what their policy and programs are for maternity hospital stays and follow-up care, and discuss any concerns you may have with your doctor.

## Questions That Can Help You Choose Your Doctor or Midwife

◆ What types of clinicians will be involved in your care? Can you choose either a doctor or a midwife? What role do nurses or nurse practitioners play?

◆ To what hospital(s) are patients admitted for labor and delivery? Does the hospital have anesthesia available twenty-four hours a day? (Research has indicated that the availability of around-the-clock on-site anesthesia services may reduce cesarean section rates.) If you have a preference for a particular hospital, you may be able to choose a doctor or midwife who will admit you there.

◆ If you have previously delivered by cesarean section, and hope to deliver vaginally this time, which clinicians are most experienced and supportive of vaginal birth after cesarean (often called "VBAC")?

◆ If you have a complicating health factor like diabetes, or are pregnant with twins or more, which doctors have the most experience with these conditions?

◆ How many doctors cover the practice? What are the odds that your doctor will deliver your baby? Who is available when your doctor isn't? How can you meet the other doctors in the practice?

◆ Can you get appointments at times that are most convenient for you?

## Things to Discuss with Your HMO Clinician

◆ Any philosophical or cultural beliefs that will influence your pregnancy and childbirth.

◆ Any religious beliefs that might affect your care during pregnancy or childbirth, including issues around the use of blood products.

◆ Your feelings about prenatal testing (like ultrasound and amniocentesis) to determine if your baby has any abnormalities.

◆ Your feelings about abortion or treatment options if prenatal testing reveals abnormalities.

◆ Your feelings about pain control and medication during labor and delivery.

◆ Whether medical school students or residents will be involved in your care at the hospital, and how you feel about that.

◆ Whether and how you would like your family included in the childbirth experience, and whether the hospital has regulations about family members attending the birth.

◆ Under what circumstances you might have a cesarean section delivery, and the risks and benefits associated with it.

◆ Whether the hospital is equipped to handle high-risk deliveries or newborns in need of intensive care, and if not, what the backup arrangements are.

◆ If your caregiver is a midwife, how her role differs from that of an obstetrician, and under what circumstances she might involve an obstetrician in your care.

◆ Prenatal and parental education classes that are available from your doctor or your HMO.

◆ Whether there are classes for older siblings to help them adjust to a new baby.

◆ Your feelings about breast versus bottle feeding, and whether the hospital staff is more supportive of one method over the other.

◆ Whether the hospital itself has policies that might impact your care (for example, if you want to have your fallopian tubes tied after delivery, a Catholic hospital might refuse your request).

◆ How long your hospital stay is likely to be, and whether you or your baby will have any follow-up care at home.

# MENTAL HEALTH
# AND SUBSTANCE ABUSE CARE

Coverage for mental illness and drug and alcohol abuse varies greatly from state to state and HMO to HMO. You may even find that your employer has "carved out" or separated your mental health and substance abuse coverage from the rest of your HMO coverage, in order to gain greater control of the cost and quality of this type of treatment. (Although the two conditions—mental illness and substance abuse—are not the same, they are often interrelated, and the way they are covered by HMOs and other insurance plans is often the same.)

The wide variation among plans reflects differences in opinion among health care professionals about what kinds of treatment are most effective, how much treatment is affordable, and whether people faced with the anxieties and troubling complexities of everyday living (sometimes called the "worried well") should be entitled to the same level of coverage as someone with serious psychiatric problems.

Since HMOs cover treatment for strep throat as well as cancer, should they also cover therapy for someone upset about the breakup of a marriage the same way they cover clinical depression? If HMOs don't take care of less serious mental problems, are they abandoning their commitment to prevention and possibly leaving their members vulnerable to more serious problems (and the HMO vulnerable to higher treatment costs) down the road? Is there any proof that long-term therapy (including psychotherapy) is more effective in treating mental and substance abuse problems than less expensive short-term therapy? Can a psychiatrist be more helpful than a psychiatric social worker? What is the relationship between illnesses of the mind and illnesses of the body? And what about inpatient treatment versus outpatient treatment? These are some of the many questions that drive the debate over appropriate care and coverage.

One successful model for HMO mental health and substance abuse care and coverage includes the following elements:

◆ Direct access by self-referral to mental health or substance abuse emergency care and crisis intervention
when and where they are needed.

◆ A professional assessment of the severity of a patient's
problems and a personal long- or short-term treatment
plan.

◆ Treatment in the most appropriate and effective setting
provided by appropriate professionals.

◆ A range of therapies that are flexible and that have been
proven to be effective.

◆ Ongoing reevaluation and adjustment of your treatment
plan.

◆ No limits in benefits for people with severe psychiatric
or substance abuse disorders; those with less severe
problems would also receive well-planned treatment but
it is not unlimited and it involves greater cost sharing.

## Understanding Your Benefits

It is very important for you to understand your HMO
mental health and substance abuse benefits and how to
gain access to them. The only way to do that is to read your
member contract carefully, and talk to your HMO or HMO
primary care doctor if there is anything you don't understand. Some of the key issues are:

◆ What is the overall treatment philosophy of your
HMO toward mental health and substance abuse, and
can it be demonstrated that it is a sound philosophy
in terms of outcomes, quality of care, and cost effectiveness?

◆ How do you get access to covered mental health or substance abuse treatment? Is there a special mental health and substance abuse phone number you are required to call?

◆ Can you make an appointment directly with your HMO's mental health and substance abuse professionals, or do you need a referral from your primary care doctor?

◆ What types of mental health and substance abuse providers are part of your HMO's network, and where are they located?

◆ Can you follow different rules to get care in an emergency or crisis, and how does your HMO define them?

◆ Will you be evaluated and have a treatment plan developed, and by whom?

◆ Are there limitations on the number of days of treatment, cost of treatment, or types of treatment available and covered?

◆ Will the cost you pay for visits differ depending on whether your therapy is individual or group, long-term or short-term?

◆ Are halfway houses covered as part of your treatment plan?

◆ Will drugs that are necessary for the treatment of psychiatric disorders be covered by your HMO, and will you have to share the cost?

◆ What services are covered for evaluation or treatment if you are away from home, traveling, or at college?

◆ Are services related to mental retardation, learning disabilities, and speech disorders covered?

Whatever the answers to these questions turn out to be, you are likely to find that the standard HMO rule applies: Except in an emergency, you should make sure your care is authorized in advance by your HMO doctor or HMO, and you should expect to get your care from your HMO's network of mental health and substance abuse providers.

## Choosing the Right Mental Health Provider

Finding the right mental health care provider is often challenging, especially for patients who are feeling less than their best emotionally. It can also be particularly difficult for patients who have already been in some form of therapy to change to a new provider when they join an HMO. Whether your needs for mental health care are new or ongoing, short- or long-term, you want to make sure your HMO mental health provider is someone you feel comfortable with.

If you have been under the care of a psychiatrist or psychologist or other mental health professional, you should check to see if he is part of the HMO network. If he is, you won't have to change providers. If he isn't, you might tell him that you would like him to be. If that isn't feasible, or is not something that could happen quickly, then you will need to choose a new caregiver who is affiliated with your HMO, or pay for continued therapy out of pocket.

Many HMOs allow patients to "self-refer" to affiliated mental health providers, which means you can call and make a mental health appointment without being referred by your HMO primary care doctor. However, you should consider your primary care doctor a good resource to help you choose a mental health provider who is suited to your needs and preferences, and in helping you get an appointment with that provider.

## Questions That Can Help You Choose Your Therapist

◆ Do you need a referral from your primary care doctor to see a mental health therapist?

◆ Will you have a choice of therapists, or will you be assigned to one?

◆ What kinds of therapists are available to you? Psychiatrists? Psychologists? Psychiatric nurses? Substance abuse counselors? Social workers? Others?

◆ Who is most experienced with your kind of issue, illness, or disorder; what is his or her training and approach to treating your kind of problem?

◆ If you have cultural, religious, or philosophical beliefs that may influence the kind of care you want, which therapist will be most supportive of them?

◆ What are the waiting times for evaluation?

◆ Which providers offer flexible appointment schedules that are most likely to meet your needs?

◆ Can you easily receive a consultation or second opinion if you disagree with the treatment recommendations or feel you are not getting better?

◆ How easily can you change therapists if you're not happy?

◆ What hospitals are used? If you have a preference, you may be able to choose a doctor who admits there.

◆ What happens in an emergency? Who is available nights and weekends?

## Things to Discuss with Your Therapist

◆ Any cultural, religious, or philosophical beliefs that may influence the kind of care you want.

◆ How your care will be coordinated if you will be receiving mental health and/or substance abuse care from more than one source, or if you have ongoing physical issues for which you will be seeing your primary care physician.

◆ Any programs or groups that focus on special issues that are of concern to you (e.g., eating disorders, sexual abuse, living with HIV).

◆ How decisions are made around long-term versus short-term therapies.

◆ What your treatment plan will be; how your progress will be assessed; how your treatment plan will be adjusted.

◆ What will happen if you disagree with your therapist's treatment plan for you.

◆ How much care is covered, and what your options are if that coverage runs out.

◆ Whether there are flexible benefits: whether you can trade inpatient days for more outpatient appointments.

◆ Whether your mental health records are integrated with your other health care records into a single medical record, or whether mental health records are kept separately. (Some patients prefer to have separate mental health records to safeguard confidentiality.)

## Finding the Right Drug or Alcohol Counselor

Drug or alcohol abuse is an individual problem with a broad impact. Its results often spread far beyond the patient to affect the lives of his or her family, friends, and coworkers. That's why it's so important to find a counselor who can provide appropriate care for the patient and advice and support for the rest of the family too.

If you are an HMO member seeking help for drug or alcohol abuse, talk first with your primary care doctor. He will be able to advise you on your next steps, including getting help to determine whether or not you have a drug or alcohol abuse problem, and can refer you to an appropriate provider within the HMO network. If you are already in a course of treatment for alcohol or substance abuse when you join the HMO, you should ask if your current provider is part of the HMO network, or if you can continue seeing him even if he's not. If the answer to either question is no, then you should try to choose the HMO provider with whom you think you will work the best.

One of the ongoing debates about substance abuse care is whether inpatient treatment is more effective than outpatient treatment. The image of celebrities retreating to a secluded treatment center for a month or so and emerging renewed and healthy fuels the impression that inpatient treatment is most effective. This is not always the case, and your HMO may have programs that provide intensive treatment and counseling on an outpatient basis. Check with your primary care provider or your substance abuse counselor to find out what the treatment options are, and what the advantages are of each.

*Questions That Can Help You Choose a Substance Abuse Counselor*

◆ Can you choose a primary substance abuse clinician who will manage all your care and treatment related to substance abuse?

◆ Which doctors have expertise about your particular type of problem?

◆ Which doctors have expertise in family intervention and support?

◆ What hospitals or treatment facilities are used? If you have a preference, you may be able to select a doctor who admits there.

◆ What other clinicians work with yours? Who else might you see for treatment?

◆ What happens in an emergency? Who is available nights and weekends?

*Things to Discuss with Your Substance Abuse Counselor*

◆ Any of your past experiences with substance abuse treatment, both positive and negative.

◆ Your expectations from the HMO and the doctor.

◆ How much time you might expect to spend in treatment, what the treatment options are, and what is covered by the HMO.

◆ The criteria for admission to an inpatient facility or out-patient program.

◆ Counseling options available to family members.

◆ How other non-HMO programs (like Alcoholics Anonymous) might be integrated into your treatment.

◆ Any other health problems you have concerns about.

# ORTHOPEDIC AND RHEUMATIC PROBLEMS: PAIN AND INJURIES OF THE MUSCLES, BONES, AND JOINTS

Orthopedic and rheumatic problems are a source of misery for many people, especially when they affect the back, or the joints of knees, elbows, hands, or feet. Treatment for a broken bone or a sprain is relatively simple and straightforward; serious joint injuries, back problems, and arthritis are not. If you're suffering from disabling pain, you want instant relief, and it can be maddening if you think your HMO or insurer is placing unnecessary barriers between you and the care you need.

It is estimated that 65 to 80 percent of all Americans suffer from some sort of back pain during their lifetime. Ten million suffer from chronic lower back pain.

Arthritis comes in over a hundred different forms, the majority of which have unknown causes, and affects half of all Americans sixty-five and older. The most common types of arthritis are osteoarthritis (sometimes known as degenerative joint disease), which generally affects the large weight-bearing joints; rheumatoid arthritis, which varies in severity but at its worst causes severe swelling and inflammation and significant pain; and gout, the most treatable form, which is most prevalent in older men.

Unfortunately, there is no single cure or treatment to relieve most orthopedic and rheumatic problems. Some of the treatment options include "body mechanics" (focusing on how you sit, lie, lift, stand, etc.), exercise, medication, stress reduction, manipulation of bones or muscles, acupuncture, and surgery (including arthroscopic surgery and joint replacement). Physical therapists, orthopedists, rheumatologists, chiropractors, osteopaths, acupuncturists, massage therapists, pain clinics, sports medicine clinics, and specialty hospitals all lay claim to some success in treating these types of problems. And increasingly sophisticated and expensive tools are available to diagnose certain problems, like CT scans and magnetic resonance imaging (MRI).

As an HMO member, you will have to work with your primary care doctor to navigate your way through this maze to the most appropriate and effective diagnosis and treatment.

With so many options available, excellent communication and trust between you and your primary care doctor are absolutely essential. In many cases, your primary care doctor can provide the care you need, but if you think you should be seeing a specialist instead, or if you want a type of care your HMO doesn't cover, there's a good chance you will be unhappy.

It's important for you to read and understand your HMO contract, which explains what kind of care or treatment is covered and what isn't. Many HMOs, for instance, don't cover chiropractic care or acupuncture, and there may be limits on coverage for physical therapy.

In order to see a specialist, you will need to be referred by your HMO primary care doctor. Since you should meet with your primary care doctor first to discuss all your health care needs anyway, this is a good opportunity to ask questions and let him or her know about any preferences you might have regarding a specialist.

## Questions to Ask Your Primary Care Doctor

- ◆ What role does your primary care doctor play in treating your problem?
- ◆ What is the process for diagnosing the cause of your pain?
- ◆ Once it is diagnosed, who will determine the course of treatment?
- ◆ Under what circumstances will you be referred to a specialist? How can you make sure that care is covered?
- ◆ What kind of specialists are available (orthopedists, rheumatologists, pain specialists, others), and who is most experienced with your particular problem?
- ◆ What level of specialists are available within specialty departments (e.g., doctors who specialize only in prob-

lems with the feet, hands, or back, or conditions like sco-
liosis or cerebral palsy)?

◆ For foot problems, will you see a podiatrist or an orthopedic surgeon?

◆ How far might you have to travel for services like physical therapy?

◆ What hospitals are used? If you have a preference, you
may want to ask for a referral to a specialist who admits
patients there.

## Things to Discuss with the Specialist

◆ Under what circumstances you might benefit from an
MRI or a CT scan. (These diagnostic tools are expensive,
so HMOs try to use them only when appropriate and
necessary; at the same time, patients like them because
they may provide a uniquely clear look at the body's
internal workings, without the radiation associated with
x-rays).

◆ Treatment options available for your problem.

◆ Pain-control options available to you.

◆ Appropriate exercise regimens that involve you in your
own healing.

◆ Written materials or videotapes that you can use for
self-help.

◆ Whether you can see a chiropractor, acupuncturist, or
other alternative caregiver, and whether the care is covered.

◆ Who might perform surgery if you require it.

◆ How to get a second opinion on a treatment plan if you
want one.

# PEDIATRIC CARE

Kids get sick. A lot. Ear infections, sore throats, upset stomachs, diarrhea, croup, chicken pox, bumps, and bruises are all part of childhood. Even if kids aren't sick, they need regular checkups and immunizations. So you and your child are likely to spend a lot of time seeing or consulting by phone with your doctor. That's why it's so important to choose your pediatrician or family practitioner carefully and thoughtfully. When you feel good about your child's doctor, chances are your child will too.

Trust is the most important element in any good doctor-patient relationship, and it is especially critical in pediatrics. Finding someone you feel you can trust, someone who will listen respectfully to your concerns, someone who welcomes your questions (even the ones you feel foolish asking), someone who you know has your child's best interest at heart, is essential to getting the best care for your child.

## Questions That Can Help You Choose Your Child's Doctor

◆ Can you interview some pediatricians or family practitioners before you select one? (This is often the best way to determine if you are comfortable with the doctor's style. Things to look for: Does the doctor project experience and confidence? Is she warm? Does she listen? Does she give good answers to your questions? If your child is present, does she interact with the child in a positive way?)

◆ Who has the most and the least patients, and why? (A full practice may indicate a popular doctor, but she may also be harder to see. Joining a newer practice may mean that it will be easier to get appointments.)

◆ What are the office hours for the practice and what are the pediatrician's practice hours?

- How is the practice organized? What other clinicians might your child see? Who covers for your child's doctor when she is not there? How can you meet the other clinicians in the practice?
- If you have special religious, philosophical, or cultural preferences that may impact the kind of care you want for your child, which pediatrician is likely to be most supportive?
- If your child has special health care needs or conditions, which pediatrician or other medical professional in the practice (nurse practitioner, for example) is most experienced with that particular issue?
- What specialists are used? How will your child have access to specialty care?
- What hospitals are used? If you have a preference, you may be able to choose a pediatrician who admits there.
- What happens in an emergency? Who is available at nights or on weekends?

## Things to Discuss with Your Child's HMO Clinician

- What kind of relationship you hope to have with the pediatrician.
- What kind of relationship you hope your child will have with the pediatrician.
- Any religious, cultural, philosophical, or family issues that will impact the kind of care you want for your child.
- Feelings or concerns you may have about immunizations or blood tests, or any other aspect of your child's care.
- If your child needs care from a specialist, how his or her care will be managed.

◆ Previous medical experiences or relationships your child has had that were strongly positive or negative, and why.

◆ Methods you and the pediatrician can use together to help overcome your child's fears and to help her establish trust in her new doctor.

◆ How you will know when your child needs regular checkups.

◆ The best way for you to get your questions answered when your child doesn't need an appointment.

◆ Whether your doctor or HMO has educational brochures or classes available on childhood health issues.

◆ Whether your doctor would especially recommend any books on dealing with common childhood illnesses or on how to raise children successfully.

## PEDIATRIC SPECIAL NEEDS

Whether your child is a newborn or a teenager, nothing is more frightening than the news that he or she has a serious disorder. Fortunately, with advances in genetic counseling and conception planning, many couples who know they are at risk for passing genetic abnormalities to their children are able to take measures prior to conception that can prevent disorders as severe as Tay-Sachs disease or brain and nervous system malformations. And because prenatal screening has become so sophisticated, many disorders can be identified during pregnancy. This enables couples to make decisions about termination and allows doctors to anticipate problems and plan for treatment either before or immediately following the birth. Some problems aren't detected until birth, especially if the baby is unexpectedly premature. Other disorders aren't discovered until the baby grows, like developmental delays and learning disabilities; and still others are caused by illnesses or injuries during childhood.

Whether your child's disorder is anticipated or unexpected, you will probably want all the information, support, care, and services you can get. A normal, healthy baby requires twenty-four-hour caring; babies with special needs require that, and more. Make sure the HMO you join has ample support systems—both medical and psychological— for parents of special needs children.

If the cause of the disorder is not immediately apparent to you or your baby's doctors, then it is important to continue to try to identify its origins, both to treat it and to help prevent its recurrence if you have more children. For this, you should ask to meet with a geneticist, who can review the family histories of both parents, help determine a cause, and aid the diagnosis. Many serious genetic diseases, like cystic fibrosis, are carried by people who are never affected by them and never know they are carriers. Often they discover this only when their child is diagnosed with the disease, the first clue that both parents are carriers. Working with your primary care pediatrician, a geneticist may be able to solve the mystery of your child's abnormality or disease. This will help you plan for future pregnancies, and can also provide your child's doctors with important clues about what to anticipate as your child grows. Children born without thumbs, for instance, are often at risk for heart disease; a geneticist may be best able to help your doctor identify these associations, as well as opportunities for prevention and active management of later problems.

Premature birth is a leading cause of pediatric problems. It can result in breathing difficulties; hearing, vision, and speech loss; dental problems; learning and developmental delays; behavioral and emotional disorders;

attention deficit disorder; or hyperactivity. Other common "special needs" arise in children with Down's syndrome, neurological disorders, autism, cerebral palsy, cystic fibrosis, fragile X syndrome, or physical deformities. Whatever your child's disorder, you should check with your HMO and/or your pediatrician to make sure you understand what kind of care, and how much care, is covered. (Some HMOs for example, don't cover therapy for developmental or speech delays if the cause is not clearly medical.)

Parents of children with special needs often want to understand every aspect of their child's disorder, and every possible outcome of each intervention or treatment. This places a burden on parents that can be greatly eased by a knowledgeable, caring, communicative pediatrician in whom parents can place complete trust. The support of a group of parents who share an understanding of the anxieties, anguish, and confusion that some special needs situations create may also be invaluable.

Choosing a pediatrician in your HMO who will manage your child's care may be simple—he or she may have already been caring for other children in your family, or for your child prior to his diagnosis—or it may take some time and consideration. Sometimes parents feel a need to change pediatricians after a wrenching diagnostic process, or after they receive upsetting news; they want to "shoot the messenger," associating the current pediatrician with a sense of disaster. For this reason, or if you feel a need to choose a pediatrician who has more experience with your child's disorder, you may want to consider switching. However, if you have had a generally satisfying relationship with your pediatrician, it may be preferable to stay with a doctor who knows you and your family, and who can be helpful in monitoring and managing the impact of your child's needs on other children in the family, and on your own health and emotional equilibrium. Maintaining the doctor-child relationship means the pediatrician can observe the child over time, and reevaluate the fit between the original diagnosis and the reality for your child. Your child's current pediatrician may also be able to limit the number of your child's tests or procedures, while a new pediatrician might feel compelled to order new tests as part of getting to understand your child.

Your child could require the care of several specialists, to whom your pediatrician should refer you. It's important that the pediatrician remain at the center of these relationships, coordinating communication and managing every aspect of your child's care. While the specialists will be concerned with their particular areas of expertise, your pediatrician will care for the whole child, including providing routine care like immunizations, which are easily overlooked when there are bigger issues to deal with.

Most important of all, parents of special needs children share with all parents the need to forge a strong partnership with their child's pediatrician, a partnership based firmly on mutual respect and trust. You and this doctor may experience together some very trying and distressing times, and together you may need to make some very difficult decisions. Finding someone who can support you and guide you through these experiences and decisions, and who can provide expert care and loving attention to your child, will be of immeasurable value to you and your family.

## Questions That Can Help You Choose Your Child's Pediatrician

◆ Who has the most experience dealing with your child's disorder?

◆ If your child will be referred to specialists, who might they be, and what will the pediatrician's role be?

◆ Does the pediatrician work in a team with other clinicians? Who else might be involved in your child's care? Who is available when the doctor isn't?

◆ Where will care for your child be provided? In the doctor's office? A hospital? At home?

◆ What hospitals are used? If you have a preference, you may be able to choose a pediatrician who admits there.

## Things to Discuss with Your Child's HMO Clinician

◆ Specific concerns or fears you have about your child.

◆ How the pediatrician plans to manage your child's care; how you hope to see it managed.

◆ How the doctor-parent relationship will work best for both of you; how decisions will be made.

◆ What to do in an emergency or in an urgent or complex situation when your primary care doctor is not available.

◆ How the child's emotional well-being will be supported.

◆ How the family's stresses can be eased.

◆ How siblings can be supported.

◆ What kind of materials or groups are available on medical and nonmedical issues, like financial planning for long-term care, life insurance, or respite care resources.

◆ What kind of care is covered, and for how long.

◆ How to plan ahead should your child's disability or disorder become more severe over time, or should you become unable to care for him or her.

## SENIOR HEALTH

Americans are living longer now than ever before. Not only that, but they are staying healthier longer. Thanks to advances in medicine and to the fact that more older Americans are exercising regularly, eating healthy diets, quitting smoking, and cutting down on drinking, studies show that disability rates among the elderly have dropped in the past several years. With 32 million Americans aged sixty-five or older, and a projected 54 million in thirty years, this trend is good news for everyone.

While some people just naturally grow old gracefully and in good health, many others need medical help to do so. This may simply take the form of regular checkups and screenings for preventive care and early detection of illness, or treatment of short- or long-term illnesses or injuries. The most common chronic conditions that affect older people range from easily treatable problems to illnesses that grow progressively more difficult to manage. In order of their prevalence, these conditions include arthritis, vision loss, hearing loss, osteoporosis, diabetes, stroke, and Alzheimer's disease. In addition to these, many older people suffer from digestive problems, incontinence, and high blood pressure, and are more susceptible to prostate or breast cancer, flu, and hypothermia (exposure that causes a dangerous drop in body temperature). Some 70 percent of elderly Americans take more than one prescription drug every day, and at least one in five elderly patients suffers from short- or long-term mental illness, usually depression or anxiety.

Daunting as this list appears, there are a great many preventive measures that may delay the onset of an illness or disease, or help you avoid it altogether. There is also effective treatment for many of these conditions, and exciting new research that promises more answers on the horizon.

If you are entering or already enjoying your "golden years," you should be prepared to pay closer attention to your health, your habits, and your schedule of routine checkups. Many HMOs recommend that adults over the age of fifty should have annual checkups, including screening tests for breast, prostate, or colorectal cancer, and assessment of blood pressure, cholesterol, and any particular health concerns or risks. If you haven't had a thorough physical exam in recent years, and you are fifty or older, consult with your doctor on his or her recommendation.

As you age, you will probably be seeing your doctor more frequently than you may have in the past. Because your health care needs may be greater, it is important that you feel comfortable with and confident in your doctor. Your primary care doctor is the central figure in your relationship with the entire medical community, especially in an HMO, where he or she provides or coordinates all the care you need. If you need specialty care, for instance, your primary care doctor will refer you to the appropriate specialist and will confer with that specialist about your treatment. Likewise, if you need to be hospitalized, or need care at home, your primary care doctor will make the arrangements and will oversee your care.

Growing older doesn't necessarily mean you need to see a doctor who specializes in geriatrics (care that focuses on the aging process). Good primary care doctors provide much of the care their older patients need. However, you should feel comfortable that your doctor will call in the appropriate specialty resources on your behalf if necessary, that he understands your needs, concerns, and lifestyle, and that he can help you make informed decisions about your care and treatment.

If you already have an HMO primary care doctor, and feel your needs are changing as you age, ask yourself (and your doctor) if he has the skills and temperament you feel you want as you grow older. If not, you might ask him to recommend a different primary care doctor, or ask other older HMO members for their recommendations. If you are new to the HMO, ask older friends in your community if they are HMO members and can recommend a primary care doctor in the HMO network. Or call the HMO's member service department to talk with a representative about choosing the right doctor.

## Questions That Can Help You Choose a Doctor

◆ Can you have a personal consultation or meeting with a doctor before you choose one? (This is often the best way to determine if you are comfortable with the doctor's style, but remember you can always switch to another HMO doctor if the first one doesn't work out.)

◆ If you have particular concerns or health problems, which doctor is most experienced in those areas?

◆ How will it be determined if you need specialty care?

◆ What specialists are used? If you are currently seeing a specialist, or have a preference for someone, you might be able to choose a primary care physician who refers to that specialist.

◆ If you have special religious, philosophical, or cultural preferences that may impact the kind of care you want, which doctor is likely to be most supportive?

◆ Which doctors have the greatest percentage of older patients?

◆ Which doctors have the most and fewest patients, and why? (A full practice may indicate a popular doctor, but it may also be harder to get a quick appointment.)

- What hospitals are used? If you have a preference, you might be able to choose a primary care doctor who admits to that hospital.
- What happens in an emergency? Who is available when the doctor isn't?

## Things to Discuss with Your HMO Clinician

- How your care will be coordinated if you have multiple health needs, or are seeing more than one doctor.
- If you are taking more than one prescription medication, who will review them all to be sure they are both necessary and safe to be taken together.
- What kind of preventive care and screenings you should be getting, and how often.
- What kind of preventive measures you should be taking yourself (lifestyle or dietary changes, self-exams).
- What kind of home care will be available if you should need it.
- Any classes, groups, or educational materials that might be available on topics of importance to you.
- In what ways you might best prepare for unforeseen needs, like long-term care, nursing home care, or hospice care.
- Advice on how to talk with your adult children or other family members about handling your affairs if you are ever unable to manage them on your own.
- How to create a living will, health care proxy, or durable power of attorney to make health care decisions should you be unable to make them on your own.

## WOMEN'S HEALTH

Women's health care used to mean getting a yearly Pap smear. Today, it is much more. It's a philosophy of caring for a woman as a whole person throughout her life, anticipating and meeting her unique health care needs in a coordinated way.

From the teenaged girl's concerns about sexuality and self-image, to the older woman's questions about estrogen and osteoporosis, women's health care needs require the attention of medical professionals who understand them in the context of a woman's life. This needn't be a specialist in women's care, but merely a caring clinician, man or woman, who is able to see that medical needs are only a part of the complex collection of issues that impact most women's lives.

Some of the most common health concerns of women at different stages of their lives include issues around sexuality and relationships: sexually transmitted diseases and AIDS; fertility and reproduction; contraception; childbirth and child care; menstrual cramps and premenstrual syndrome; menopause and estrogen therapy; breast cancer and breast implants; vaginal infections and cervical cancer; anxiety, depression, and abuse. No single doctor can specialize in all of these areas; most clinicians who care for women do, in fact, rely on specialists in the course of treating their patients' various needs. Some of these specialists are exclusive to women, like gynecologists or obstetricians, and some are not (like oncologists for breast cancer or orthopedists for osteoporosis). Some HMOs have women's health clinics or special programs focusing on menopause or breast disease. For many women, this is an appealing and comfortable way to learn about their health and receive care in a coordinated, supportive fashion. Check with your HMO to see what is available.

Many women prefer to see a gynecologist as their primary care physician; some HMOs allow this. If yours doesn't, your primary care physician or a nurse practitioner who is trained in routine gynecology will probably provide your gynecological care, and will refer you to specialists for more complex issues. Your primary care physician is in the best position to get to know you as a person and understand some of the issues in your life that may affect your mental or physical health. By learning about you and your needs over time, and by coordinating and consulting with various specialists when needed, he or she should be able to provide the kind of care that is typically called women's health care.

## Questions That Can Help You Choose a Doctor

◆ Who will provide your routine gynecological care? Your primary care doctor? A gynecologist? A nurse practitioner or nurse midwife?

◆ Are there any primary care doctors in the HMO network who specialize in women's health care?

◆ Can you interview some doctors before you select one? (This is often the best way to determine if you are comfortable with the doctor's style.)

◆ If you have particular concerns or health problems, which doctors are most experienced in these areas?

◆ If you have special religious, philosophical, or cultural preferences that may impact the kind of care you want, which doctors are likely to be most supportive?

◆ Which doctors have the most and fewest patients, and why? Will that affect your ability to get an appointment when you want one?

◆ What specialists are used? If you have a preference, you might be able to choose a primary care physician who refers to that specialist. How is your care coordinated when a specialist is needed?

◆ What hospitals are used? If you have a preference, you might be able to choose a primary care physician who admits to that hospital.

## Things to Discuss with Your HMO Clinician

◆ If you are seeing more than one doctor, how your care will be  coordinated.

◆ Any classes, groups, or educational materials that might be available about women's health issues in general, or specific conditions or concerns you may have.

◆ What kind of preventive care (screenings like Pap smears or mammograms) you should be getting, and how often.

◆ What kind of preventive measures you should be taking yourself (like breast self-examination).

◆ What might happen if you want a mammogram or Pap smear, and your HMO's protocols suggest you don't need one.

◆ Any cultural, religious, or philosophical issues that might impact the kind of care you want.

◆ What kind of relationship you hope to have with your doctor.

◆ How you would like to go about making decisions about your care, especially on difficult or controversial issues like having a mastectomy versus lumpectomy to treat breast cancer, or taking hormonal replacement therapy following a hysterectomy.

## Roles and Responsibilities for Better Health Care

As an HMO member, you are entitled to a wide range of benefits, which are guaranteed in your contract if you follow the rules and requirements of your HMO. You should also consider yourself entitled to health care that is just as personal and caring and high quality as what you could receive with any other type of health insurance. But good care is not guaranteed in your contract; it requires you and your HMO doctor and your HMO to accept some important roles and responsibilities.

**YOUR ROLE**

As a consumer, a patient, and an HMO member, you should:

- Understand what you need to do in order to get health care or medical assistance—routine, urgent, or in an emergency, day or night, at home, or when you are traveling—and follow those policies and procedures at all times.
- Make sure other members of your family also understand what to do in any of these circumstances, especially children who are covered and who are away at school.
- Understand what is covered by your HMO's benefits, and what is not, by making sure you keep and review your HMO member contract.
- Understand your HMO's approach to preventive care and healthy behaviors, recognize your responsibility for your own health and safety, and follow their guidelines and recommendations as much as possible.
- Know where to get advice, information, or assistance at any time, day or night.
- Ask questions about your care and your coverage, and listen with an open mind.
- Provide your doctor with complete and accurate information about your symptoms and your health history, with the understanding that this information will be kept strictly confidential.

- Tell your doctor about the "root cause" of any medical concerns you may have. For instance, if you have had persistent pain and you want a high-tech cancer test because you read about it in the newspaper and you have a friend who had that kind of cancer, say so. This will help your doctor address the problem more directly and efficiently by understanding what is really of concern to you.
- Follow treatment plans that you and your doctor have agreed upon, and let your doctor know if you have problems or concerns about your progress.
- Use your HMO's medical services responsibly and respectfully, recognizing that you and other HMO members are sharing limited resources.
- Accept responsibility for the outcomes of your decisions about your health care.
- Speak up immediately about any concerns you have regarding the quality of health care you are receiving—to your doctor, or if that makes you uncomfortable, to your HMO's member service department. If you are still not satisfied, talk to your employer's health benefits administrator or your state's HMO regulatory agency.
- Let your HMO know immediately about any changes in your address, phone number, or your family situation (marriage, divorce, birth, or death of a family member) so they can reach you if they need to.

## YOUR DOCTOR'S ROLE

As participants in HMOs, doctors should:

- Understand the policies and procedures that HMO members need to follow to get the care they need, and help their HMO patients understand and use them.
- Ensure that patients with urgent medical problems can get the advice or treatment they need within a few hours, day or night, seven days a week.

- Provide complete and understandable information about diagnosis, treatment, and anticipated or possible outcomes, and encourage their patients to ask questions.
- When there is more than one treatment option available, explain the advantages and disadvantages of each and involve their patients in the decision-making.
- Demonstrate an understanding of, and interest in each patient, by listening and building a relationship of trust and respect.
- Provide appropriate referrals, authorization, and arrangements for specialty and hospital care; explain to patients why such care is necessary or not necessary; and provide appropriate coordination, management, and follow-up to that care.
- Be aware of the HMO's guidelines and standards for preventive care and healthy behaviors and use them to inform, counsel, and encourage members to take responsibility for their own health.

**YOUR HMO'S ROLE**

As a partner in your good health, your HMO should:

- Communicate clearly to each member about what is covered and what rules, policies, and procedures members should follow in order to receive high-quality care when and where it is needed.
- Provide easy access for members to ask questions, file complaints, or appeal decisions, and ensure follow-up and a response to member complaints or concerns.
- Help ensure that you can choose a personal primary care HMO doctor with whom you are comfortable and on whom you can rely for good health care.
- Actively encourage appropriate preventive practices and healthy behaviors for each member.
- Maintain a network of specialists, hospitals, and other

medical resources that are adequate to meet the needs of members for access to care.

- Make sure members and doctors understand how to get authorized referrals to specialists, hospitals, and other medical resources.
- Ensure that HMO members have twenty-four-hour-a-day, seven-day-a-week access to urgent and emergency care.
- Monitor, measure, and report on health care quality and patient satisfaction as well as cost.
- Remove bureaucratic barriers that could prevent patients from getting the care and service they need.
- Communicate with patients about any changes in coverage or policies that affect HMO membership, benefits, or the way they receive care.

This list of roles and responsibilities is by no means complete. For instance, members, doctors, and HMOs all have important financial responsibilities that hold the partnership together. Check your HMO's new-member guide and contract for other "rights and responsibilities." As you learn more about your HMO membership, you may want to add to the list.

# 8

## Problems and Complaints: A Primer for Taking Action

Your health and your money. For most of us, there are few things that are more personal, more important, or more capable of making us very happy . . . or miserable. Since HMO membership, or any kind of health care coverage, for that matter, involves both your health and your money, it can be very aggravating when something goes wrong. And since HMOs make you follow rules that may be unfamiliar, the potential for confusion and frustration is even greater. You can help yourself avoid most problems if you:

- ◆ Understand your own needs and the options that are available to you.
- ◆ Understand how HMOs work and how your HMO membership will be different from what you have been used to.
- ◆ Make smart choices about your HMO and your doctor.
- ◆ Get a good start with your membership.
- ◆ Become well informed about your benefits and your HMO's coverage rules.
- ◆ Become an active participant with your doctor in decisions about your health care.

According to public opinion surveys, most HMO members say they are satisfied with their plans, but you need to know what to do if you are not. You need to be ready and willing to act. And HMOs, unlike most traditional health insurance plans, have formal procedures, detailed in your member contract, that you can use to complain, file a grievance, or appeal a decision about your care or coverage.

## HOW WILL YOU REACT TO A PROBLEM?

Unhappy consumers come in all types: they can be active, passive, aggressive, gently persuasive, angry, conciliatory, bullying. Most of us find it a lot easier to complain to our family and friends about what bothers us than to do something about it. And by the time a problem gets so bad that we are willing to act, we are about to explode. This certainly doesn't make for easy or constructive communication with someone we expect to solve our problem.

What do you do if you go to a nice restaurant and the food is overcooked? How do you deal with a car repair shop that keeps finding new problems without solving the one you came in for? What if the mail-order sweater you bought for your spouse's birthday is two weeks overdue? How we react to these types of situations has a lot to do with our personalities, how seriously we take the problem, whether we think we share the blame, and how inconvenient it will be to act on our rights as a consumer. The same is true for health care. With your HMO, you have very important rights as a member and very specific steps you can take to make sure you get what you deserve.

Detailed descriptions of your rights as an HMO member can usually be found in two places, in your member contract and in a separate document that specifically lists member or patient rights. It is very important that you read and keep both of these documents, because if a problem does come up, they will give you the facts you need to communicate clearly to your doctor or HMO about what you are entitled to and what you intend to do about it.

## SPEAKING UP

If you have strong opinions about the care, service, or coverage you receive from your HMO or your doctor, speak up. Be as specific as possible, whether your feelings are positive or negative. Always indicate whether or not you expect a response. This kind of feedback can be very useful to your HMO, both to encourage good care and service and to help point out problems, and it should be welcomed. Let your HMO know if:

- ◆ Someone in the enrollment department solved your problem without making you do the work.
- ◆ You liked the way your daughter's pediatrician helped get her ready for a difficult blood test.
- ◆ You have trouble getting through on the phone.
- ◆ You don't mind waiting for your appointment, but you think someone should tell you the reason for the delay.
- ◆ You think your HMO needs to do a better job of reporting on the results of lab tests.
- ◆ You are upset about an increase in your office visit copayments.
- ◆ English is not your first language and you want your HMO to hire more staff members who speak your language.

If you have a serious complaint about your coverage or the quality of your medical care, or you feel you are getting bad service or are being mistreated or ignored by someone who should be helping you, you can formally complain. In many cases, you can start with your doctor or with someone in the department where you are having problems. If you're clear about what bothers you, you can often clear up a problem very quickly. (Remember, if you disagree with your doctor's diagnosis or recommendation for treatment, you can seek a medical second opinion within the rules of your HMO, or pay for one yourself.)

If you are uncomfortable about complaining to your doctor, you should call or write to your HMO's member service department, which is responsible for providing information and handling complaints. You may also find that your HMO doctor's office, health center, or clinic has a member advisor or consumer advocate on site to whom you can talk.

All complaints, whether they are over the phone or in writing, should be responded to by your HMO unless you tell them you don't expect a response. Ideally, they should be resolved to your satisfaction. If not, you should be told how you can file a formal complaint or a grievance. When you file either of these, you should be notified by your HMO that it is being investigated, and you should receive a response within a reasonable amount of time from a responsible manager of your HMO. Your contract will explain these procedures in detail. You might file a complaint if:

◆ You have been getting bills and notices from a collection agency for a hospital visit that was supposed to be covered, and you are concerned about your credit rating.

◆ You were told that you had been referred to a specialist for five visits, but your HMO cut off your coverage after three.

◆ Your mammogram found an unusual mass and you think it is taking much too long to get a follow-up appointment with an HMO specialist.

## MEMBER APPEALS

If you disagree with your HMO's refusal to cover services you think you need, or with its refusal to pay for services that you have already received (they deny a claim), you can formally appeal a coverage decision. A member appeal is a formal process that will be described in your member contract. Check to see if there is a time limit that requires you to file an appeal within a certain period after the decision with which you disagree.

Your appeal will be sent to a committee that could include HMO members, and you may be given the chance to attend a meeting or hearing at which your case will be discussed. If your appeal involves your medical care, you will have to grant permission for the committee to review your medical records. Its approval or denial of your appeal will be communicated to you in writing, and it should tell you the exact reasons for the decision.

HMOs can take weeks to make a final decision on an appeal, so if you think that serious medical harm could result from a delay in getting the medical services you want to have covered, you should ask if there is a way you can get an immediate decision. In some HMOs, the medical director or some other high-level medical administrator has the authority to bypass the appeals process and decide on your case.

If your appeal is denied and you still disagree with your HMO's decision, you should be able to take it another step, to an outside third party, like an arbitration service or a state regulatory agency. Check your member contract. You might appeal to your HMO, if:

◆ You took your child to an emergency room when he fell on some rocks and cut his head open, but your HMO won't cover it because they decided it was not a life-threatening emergency.

◆ You need delicate brain surgery and you have been told that the hospital your HMO will send you to is not as good as another one in the same city; you know they cost about the same and you would be willing to pay any difference yourself.

◆ Your HMO refuses to cover a new cancer treatment that it says is experimental and you want the decision formally reconsidered.

◆ Your HMO's marketing brochure said they cover podiatric care, but now they won't pay for the procedures your podiatrist recommends.

There is no guarantee that your appeal will be decided in your favor in any one of these cases, but if you think you are being denied care or coverage unfairly and that you have good evidence to support your point of view, it's the best way to get a fair hearing. Some of the factors that will be considered in your appeal include: whether or not you followed the requirements of your HMO member contract; whether you made a good-faith effort to follow the rules; whether following the HMO's rules might have placed your life or health in jeopardy; whether the way the HMO interpreted its requirements were unreasonable or arbitrary.

## OTHER PLACES TO TURN FOR HELP

Finally, there are other outside parties that can be advocates for you. Your employer's health benefits department should be willing to go to bat, since they probably pay a big part of the bill. Members of some labor unions can turn to their health and welfare trust funds for help. If you are enrolled through Medicare or Medicaid, you can contact the federal or state agencies responsible for those programs. You can bring your case to the attention of your state's insurance department, consumer protection agency, or public health department if you feel you aren't being treated fairly. If you think you are being ignored by your HMO or by the regulators, a call or letter to your state legislator or member of Congress is very likely to get someone to pay attention to you. And if you have been the victim of fraud, breach of contract, or medical malpractice, you can pursue legal action on your own.

## WHO OWNS YOUR PROBLEM?

Often, the best way to get a complaint resolved or a problem solved is by making sure someone owns it. We've all experienced situations in which we get bounced around on the phone from department to department, or where someone says he will "take care of it," but we never hear from him again. Then there's the opposite experience, when something clicks and you know that the person on the phone has taken full responsibility for dealing with your complaint, that he'll personally go the extra mile to respond to your concerns. Here are some ways to encourage someone to own your problem.

◆ Begin by letting the person you speak to know—as calmly and clearly as possible—how frightened, upset, or frustrated you are, and why.

◆ State your problem as clearly and simply as possible and ask if the person you are talking to is the right person to solve your problem and, if not, who you should talk to.

◆ If you speak by phone to a staff person at your doctor's office, your HMO's member service department or claims department, or at an outside agency, write down his or her name and phone number, the time when you called, the questions you asked, and the answers you got.

◆ If your doctor says she will help you with a medical concern, ask, "Does that mean you are taking responsibility for solving my problem?"

◆ If your doctor has a nurse or assistant you have a good relationship with, ask her the same question.

◆ In addition to asking if the person you talk to will take responsibility for your problem, ask what he or she will do next, if there is anything you need to do, and when you can expect to get your problem solved.

◆ Treat the person you talk to like a friend and an ally, not an enemy, and be very clear and detailed about what your problem is, how it is affecting you, and what you hope the outcome will be.

## SWITCHING DOCTORS

If you're having problems with your HMO, it may have nothing to do with coverage rules or administrative systems. It may be that you feel uncomfortable with the quality of care or service you are getting from your HMO doctor. Sometimes the chemistry just doesn't work for you. This doesn't mean you should switch doctors without trying to resolve your problem or complaint. You may find that the problem is one of miscommunication and that your doctor is anxious to satisfy your needs. If your problem is with an HMO specialist, you may be able to get a different referral from your primary care doctor. You have to do your part to make sure you are clear about your concerns. Like any relationship, yours with your doctor takes time and it takes effort. But you should never feel trapped or intimidated into maintaining a relationship that does not work for you.

If you decide you want to switch doctors, you should be able to do so without confronting the doctor or the doctor's staff. There is no reason for you to feel uncomfortable about your choice. Your HMO's member service or consumer relations department should make the arrangements for you or tell you how. It might be helpful to tell the person who makes the arrangements why you decided to switch doctors. Explain what you found uncomfortable in your relationship with your former doctor and what you are looking for in your relationship with your new doctor. By sharing your expectations, you'll increase your chances of making a choice that meets your needs this time around.

Note: If you switch primary care doctors and your previous doctor had referred you to a specialist, it's possible that you'll have to switch specialists as well (if your new doctor uses different referral specialists). Even if you are able to stay with the same specialist, your new primary care doctor will probably have to authorize a new referral. Ask the person who helps you switch doctors to help you make the arrangements for your new specialty referral at the same time.

### CASE EXAMPLE:
#### WHEN YOU THINK IT'S TIME TO SWITCH DOCTORS

*Jan had been an HMO member for almost a year, and she had been so healthy she hadn't had a single appointment with her primary care doctor until very recently. A few months ago, she started having serious stomach pains. She had trouble eating and was losing sleep. She finally decided to see her HMO doctor, and after a brief exam, she was told that there was nothing seriously wrong. Her doctor blamed stress and recommended an over-the-counter medicine.*

*Jan's problem got worse, and she scheduled another appointment, which was even more aggravating to her than the first. She assumed her doctor would recommend some tests or have her see a specialist, but she didn't. Jan came away feeling that her doctor wasn't listening to her and that she wasn't being taken seriously. When she had lost her temper, her doctor had said, "What do you expect? You belong to an HMO, you know!" A friend at work reminded Jan that her company's open enrollment period was coming up, and suggested that it might be time to bail out of the HMO. What should Jan do?*

*There were some earlier steps Jan could have taken that might have helped her avoid the problem. If she had met with her doctor or scheduled a routine appointment sometime in the first few months of her membership, she would have been able to get a sense of how well they could communicate and how comfortable she felt with her approach to care. When she became ill, she should have made sure she was fully prepared before her appointment: that she brought the right information to her appointment and asked the right questions. But now it's too late for that. So she has several options:*

◆ *She could ask for a second opinion. If Jan's doctor resists, she could call her HMO's member service department.*

◆ *She could switch doctors, which she should be able to do quickly. Chances are, a friend or coworker could recommend another HMO primary care doctor she would feel more comfortable with. She might not get a different diagnosis or treatment, but she could get a fresh start and try to establish a relationship of trust with her new doctor.*

*She decided to start by calling her HMO's member service department to tell them about her doctor's comment "What do you expect?" She made it clear that what she expected was to receive the care she needed, to be treated with respect, and to get a clear explanation of what her doctor was recommending and why. Her complaint received a quick response in the form of an offer to sign her up with a new primary care doctor.*

*Jan decided that the problem was probably the doctor, not the HMO, so she chose a new doctor, recommended by several friends, whom she found much easier to talk with. As it turned out, however, her doctor recommended that she switch to another HMO in which he participated, and which he felt was much more committed to quality of care, so when her employer had its open enrollment period, she did.*

## SWITCHING HEALTH PLANS

Sometimes things still don't work out. You may find that belonging to an HMO is really not right for you, or that the HMO you have joined is not a good fit, considering what is most important to you. If the opportunity is available to you, it may be time to switch.

The number one reason people switch health care coverage these days is that they have to: they don't have a choice in the matter. In other words, the health plan they have belonged to is no longer available to them because they have changed jobs or moved, or their employer has decided not to offer it anymore. This last reason, an employer decision, is becoming more and more common as employers look for ways to control their health benefits costs. For people who switch voluntarily, the top reason is cost. Dissatisfaction with benefits, quality, and access to care are other typical reasons.

If you are covered for health care through your employer, you will probably have a chance to switch plans once a year at the "open enrollment period." If you have nongroup, Medicare, or Medicaid coverage, different rules may apply, so check with your HMO or the sponsoring government agency for details.

When the time comes to switch, you will want to choose your new health plan, whether it is an HMO or not, with care. Start by writing down what you like and don't like about your current plan. Then, for everything you are seriously dissatisfied with, write down what could make you satisfied. This will give you another chance to consider whether there are some issues that could be worked out with your current plan that would help you avoid switching. It also gives you a checklist of questions to ask about any new plans you are considering.

If you are unhappy with the cost of your current plan, make sure the total costs for a new plan will be less. If you have been dissatisfied with your benefits, the quality of care, or access, make sure a new plan will treat you differently. If you hate your HMO but love your doctor, make sure you know whether you will be able to continue to see him or her, and don't hesitate to ask for advice. In other words, go back to the beginning of this book and start again, with a clear understanding of your needs and your expectations. Then do what's necessary to find the right health plan for you, and to get the most out of it for your good health and peace of mind.

# 9

## Staying Healthy:
## Recommended Screening Tests
## and Guidelines for Healthy Living

HMOs are designed to keep you as healthy as possible, by preventing disease, catching problems at their earliest stages, and using appropriate treatment to restore you to good health. Prevention works, but you have to be an active participant. The following advice on screening tests and vaccinations, along with tips on healthy behaviors, were developed by the physicians of Harvard Community Health Plan. They are intended to be guidelines, not medical advice that applies to everyone, so you should discuss your specific preventive care needs, and those of other members of your family, with your own doctor.

### SCREENING TESTS

Screening tests are designed to identify problems in people who may have a particular disease. This means some healthy people will test positive, but after further testing most won't prove to have the disease. It's important to have all necessary follow-up tests done, however, so that any medical problems that are diagnosed will get proper treatment.

When detected early, many cancers can be cured, and conditions like high blood pressure can be treated before they create other medical problems.

## Screening Tests for Adults

Recommended periodic screening tests for adults include:

- A routine health assessment
- Stool screening for signs of colon cancer
- Blood pressure measurement for hypertension (high blood pressure)
- A cholesterol test to detect risk of heart attack or stroke
- Tuberculosis screening test
- Breast exam for lumps that might be breast disease
- Mammogram to detect possible breast cancer
- Pap smear to detect precancerous irregularities or cancer in the cervix
- Testicular exam to detect lumps that might be testicular cancer
- Prostate exam to detect signs of prostate cancer

## Screening Tests for Children

Periodic screening tests help pediatricians diagnose childhood medical problems early, when they are easiest to treat. They include:

- Tuberculosis screening test
- Urinalysis
- Blood count
- Lead screening
- Vision screening
- Hearing screening

# VACCINES

Some vaccines should be given to everyone, starting soon after birth; others are most helpful to people likely to be exposed to, or endangered by, a particular illness. The most important vaccines of both types include:

- ◆ DTP (diphtheria, tetanus, pertussis)
- ◆ TD (tetanus-diphtheria booster)
- ◆ OPV (polio)
- ◆ MMR (measles, mumps, rubella)
- ◆ Hib-conjugate (hemophilus influenza type B)
- ◆ Hepatitis B
- ◆ Influenza (flu)
- ◆ Pneumococcal pneumonia

(Please see "Screening and Immunization Guidelines" appendix on page 227 for more information.)

# HEALTH AND SAFETY

Good health can result from a partnership between you and your health care team. By adopting healthy habits, you can cut down your risk of serious illness and are likely to enjoy a longer, more active life.

## Tobacco

It's no secret that smoking endangers your health. Even smokeless tobacco—like snuff or chewing tobacco—isn't harmless. Some of the illnesses associated with tobacco include:

- ◆ Increased risk of lung, throat, mouth, and bladder cancers.

◆ Increased risk of emphysema, which destroys lung tissue and makes breathing very difficult.

◆ Higher risks of stroke and high blood pressure, and, for women, miscarriage and low-birthweight babies.

◆ Harm from secondhand smoke, especially to children of smokers, who are more likely to suffer from colds, flu, pneumonia, and sudden infant death syndrome (SIDS) than children of nonsmokers, and to people with asthma or other breathing problems.

To improve your chances of becoming a successful quitter:

◆ Talk to your clinician about programs to help you quit and ask if you might benefit from nicotine gum or the nicotine patch to help control withdrawal symptoms.

◆ Write down why, where, and when you smoke and all your reasons for wanting to quit. Enlist support from friends and coworkers and develop new activities for times when you used to smoke.

◆ Exercise to relieve withdrawal symptoms. Celebrate a smokeless day with a small reward, and mark smokeless weeks with something bigger.

## Alcohol and Drug Abuse

Substance abuse touches people at every level of society. While many of us enjoy relaxing with an occasional drink, drinking spins out of control for one in five Americans. Long-term alcohol abuse damages vital organs like the liver, brain, and kidneys, and reduces life expectancy by ten to twenty years.

Illegal drugs such as crack, heroin, and marijuana may also take a heavy toll on the body. And blood-borne diseases like AIDS and hepatitis B are spread by people sharing needles to inject any drug, including steroids.

In adolescents and young adults, substance abuse is linked to half the deaths caused by motor vehicle accidents, injuries, homicides, and suicides. Babies whose mothers used alcohol or drugs while pregnant often have birth defects and physical, emotional, and developmental problems. Finally, alcohol and drug abuse can take a personal toll, from ruined relationships to lost jobs and opportunities.

Breaking addictive patterns—whether problem drinking or dependence on other drugs—isn't easy, but it can be done. If you answer "yes" to any of the following questions, seek help by calling your doctor or other HMO clinician for counseling and a referral to an appropriate support group, or for information on self-help groups like Alcoholics Anonymous and Narcotics Anonymous.

- ◆ Have you ever felt a need to cut down on your use of alcohol or drugs?
- ◆ Do you ever feel guilty about substance abuse or the way you act under the influence of alcohol or drugs?
- ◆ Have you ever felt annoyed at a spouse, friend, coworker, or anyone else for criticizing your use of alcohol or drugs?
- ◆ Is drinking or drug use jeopardizing your job, causing financial difficulties, or affecting your relationships?

## Cardiovascular Health

The heart and a system of blood vessels that travel through the body form the cardiovascular system. Excess weight, inactivity, high blood pressure, and blood vessels narrowed by cholesterol deposits contribute to heart attacks and strokes, two major causes of sickness and death.

A good recipe for cardiovascular health is to keep cholesterol and blood pressure within normal limits, eat a diet with no more than 30 percent fat—20 percent or less is even better—and exercise regularly. These goals are closely entwined. Cutting dietary fat often lowers the cholesterol count, and frequent aerobic exercise strengthens the heart muscle, strips away pounds, and helps maintain blood pressure at a healthy level.

►Talk to your doctor or other HMO clinician about diet and exercise options that can improve your health. Then set up weekly and monthly goals, and reward yourself for meeting them.

►Understand and use the nutrition labels on food. Steer clear of products with a high percentage of saturated fats. Eat more vegetables and grains, and choose fruit for dessert. Ask for dressings and sauces "on the side," so you can decide how much to use.

►Talk with an HMO clinician about starting a new exercise program. Plan three or more exercise sessions a week for at least twenty minutes each. Biking, swimming, roller-skating, cross-country skiing and—easiest of all—walking are excellent choices. Varying activities will add to your enjoyment. Add exercise into your daily routine: Walk to work (or at least park your car at a distance) and use the stairs instead of an elevator.

## Sexual Activity

While sexual activity is a healthy, pleasurable part of life, some behaviors are dangerous. Each year, more than six million new cases of sexually transmitted diseases (STDs), like gonorrhea, chlamydia, and herpes, are counted among teens and adults. Untreated STDs can damage the nervous system, liver, and reproductive organs. And the viruses that cause AIDS and hepatitis B can be passed on in body fluids, such as semen and vaginal fluids, during unprotected sex.

Teenage pregnancies, which can cause health problems in mothers and low birthweight in babies, affect well over one million girls annually. Low-birthweight babies are more vulnerable to illness than babies of normal weight, and may have long-term difficulties, such as learning and behavior problems.

◆ To prevent unwanted pregnancies, abstain from sex or use effective contraception. Discuss birth control with your doctor or nurse practitioner.

◆ Latex condoms combined with a spermicide containing nonoxynol-9 offer good protection against AIDS and other sexually transmitted diseases when used properly and consistently.

◆ If you are sexually active and have had several partners or think you have an STD, ask your clinician about the need for STD screening tests.

◆ Call the National AIDS/HIV Hotline at (800) 342-AIDS for free educational materials written for children or adults explaining AIDS, HIV, and safe sex, or ask your clinician for information on AIDS and HIV. For publications explaining sexually transmitted diseases, call the National STD Hotline at (800) 227-8922.

## Stress

Snarled-up traffic, looming deadlines, and even happy events like a wished-for baby or a new home cause stress. When meeting such challenges, your muscles tense, breathing quickens, and adrenaline spills into the bloodstream, creating a surge of energy. Feelings of anxiety, fear, or anger can result.

A pileup of daily pressures can push your body into an almost continuous state of alert, which may be associated with physical symptoms like frequent headaches and insomnia. Some studies suggest a connection between stress and ulcers, irritable bowel syndrome, high blood pressure, and heart attacks. Certainly stress affects the quality of life, and in some cases encourages people to turn to alcohol or drugs for relief.

While you can't always control life events, you can learn useful methods to cope:

◆ Set limits when juggling work, home life, and social plans. Learn to say no to excessive demands at work and in your personal life.

◆ Build short breaks into busy days to allow your body a chance to unwind.

◆ Take up meditation, t'ai chi, yoga, or other activities that encourage relaxation. (Your HMO may offer courses or discounts on courses.) Physical exercise is a great stress reducer.

◆ Ask your doctor or other HMO clinician for advice on how to deal with stress.

## Safety

Millions of injuries and deaths are caused each year by motor vehicle and bicycling accidents, choking, poisoning, fires, and household hazards. Every age has its dangers: small objects put in the mouth may harm a toddler; sports or motor vehicle accidents can leave older children, teens, and adults banged up or worse; and a loose rug or an inadequate eyeglass prescription can be a threat to people who are elderly or disabled. Fortunately, you can do a lot to prevent accidents:

◆ Ask your HMO doctor or other clinician for age-appropriate publications on safety, including fire precautions, childproofing your home, and bicycle safety.

◆ Wear seatbelts and use infant and child safety seats whenever you're in a car.

◆ Do a home safety check. List what needs to be done and fix the most worrisome items first. Often, simple changes—like turning pot handles toward the back of the stove, where toddlers can't reach them—can make a big difference.

◆ Bikes and roller skates may provide hours of safe fun if you follow traffic safety rules and wear proper equipment for the sport, such as well-fitting helmets and elbow and knee pads.

◆ Sign a family pact for safety. For a teenager, that might include a contract asking for parental car service after a party if the teen—or a friend who's driving—has been drinking. For all family members, it could include practicing fire-escape routes and keeping poison-control and other emergency numbers by the phone.

# Screening and Immunization Guidelines

One of the nation's largest HMOs, Harvard Community Health Plan, recommends regularly scheduled screening tests and immunizations for all of its members. Starting at birth and continuing at regular intervals through adulthood, they are effective in detecting or preventing certain diseases in the majority of people.

These preventive-care guidelines were developed by Harvard Community Health Plan physicians, who regularly evaluate the scientific evidence as well as general guidelines prepared by national panels of experts. They don't recommend that all screenings take place each year.

You should talk to your own primary care physician at your next regularly scheduled exam about any tests that are overdue. If you don't expect to have a check-up or a doctor's visit within the next year, call your doctor's office to discuss scheduling the needed tests.

## CHILDREN

|  |  | Frequency | | | |
|---|---|---|---|---|---|
| procedure | for | 0–23 months | 2–6 years | 7–12 years | 13–17 years |

### screening tests

| routine check-up | general health | by 4 weeks; and 2, 4, 6, 9, 12, 15, and 18 months | every year | every 2 years | every 1–2 years |
| TB screening test | tuberculosis | once between 9 and 15 months | once between 3 and 5 years | | once between 13 and 16 years |
| blood test[1] | anemia | once between 9 and 12 months | | | once for girls |
| lead screening | lead poisoning | 12 months | 2, 3, and 4 years (more frequently if at increased risk); yearly until age 6 in RI | | |
| urinalysis[1] | infection, kidney disease, diabetes | | once between 3 and 4 years | | |
| visual acuity | clarity of vision | | 4 years, once between 5 and 6 years | every | 2 years |
| hearing screening with audiometer | sharpness of hearing | | once between 4 and 5 years | | once |
| breast exam[2] | breast cancer | | | | teach breast self-exam for girls 16+ |

F r e q u e n c y

| procedure | for | 0–23 months | 2–6 years | 7–12 years | 13–17 years |
|---|---|---|---|---|---|
| testicular[2] exam | testicular cancer | | | | teach testicular self-exam for boys 16+ |

## vaccines

| | | | | | |
|---|---|---|---|---|---|
| DTP | diphtheria, tetanus, pertussis | 2, 4, 6, and 15 or 18 months | once between 4 and 6 years | | |
| TD | tetanus and diphtheria | | | | once between 14 and 16 years |
| Hepatitis B[3] | hepatitis B | within a few days of birth; once between 1 and 2 months; and once between 6 and 18 months | | | |
| Hib-conjugate | haemophilus influenzae type B | 2, 4, 6, and 15 months | | | |
| OPV | polio | 2, 4, and 18 months | once between 4 and 6 years | | |
| MMR | measles, mumps, rubella | 15 months | | once between 10 and 12 years | |

1. Routine screening may be more frequent at the discretion of the primary care provider.
2. At all routine check-ups.
3. For children born after January 1, 1992.

## ADULTS

| | | Frequency | | |
| --- | --- | --- | --- | --- |
| procedure | for | 18–39 years | 40–49 years | 50+years |

### screening tests

| | | | | |
| --- | --- | --- | --- | --- |
| routine check-up | general health | every 5 years | every 1–2 years | every year |
| stool screening | colorectal cancer | —— not routinely indicated —— | | every year |
| blood pressure | hypertension | (every year at check-up or during visit to clinician for other reason) | | |
| cholesterol test | level of blood cholesterol | ———————— every 5 years ———————— | | |
| TB | tuberculosis | once if at risk[1] and not known to be positive | | |

### vaccines

| | | | | |
| --- | --- | --- | --- | --- |
| influenza | | ———— every year if at high risk[2] ———— | | every year 65 or older |
| pneumo– coccal | pneumococcal pneumonia | ———— once it at risk[3] ———— | | or at age 65 if not vaccinated previously |
| TD (booster) | tetanus and diphtheria | ———— every 10 years ———— | | |
| MMR | measles, mumps, rubella | upon entry to college if have not received two measles vaccines | | |

| procedure | for | Frequency | | |
|---|---|---|---|---|
| | | 18–39 years | 40–49 years | 50+years |

## FEMALES

| breast exam | breast cancer | every 1–2 years ——— every year ——— | | |
|---|---|---|---|---|
| mammo-gram | breast cancer | not routinely indicated | every 1–2 years | every year |
| pap smear | cervical cancer | ——————— every 1–2 years ——— | | |
| rubella immunization | rubella | vaccinate if not immune | | |

## MALES

| testicular exam | testicular cancer | at routine check-up | not routinely indicated | |
|---|---|---|---|---|
| prostate exam | prostate cancer | | | digital rectal exam at routine check-up: discuss blood screening with clinician |

1. At high risk for tuberculosis: recent immigrants from Asia, Africa, Pacific Islands, Latin America; individuals in contact with persons known to have TB; workers in health-care or correctional institutions; residents in nursing homes; individuals with a history of alcohol abuse, chronic steriod use, silicosis, malignancy or immunosuppression.

2. At high risk for influenza: individuals over age 65; individuals with chronic heart or lung disease, history of diabetes, kidney disease, immunosuppression; nursing-home residents; health care workers.

3. At high risk for pneumococcal pneumonia: same as influenza; also individuals who have had spleen surgically removed or who have splenic dysfunction (as in sickle-cell disease).

# A Glossary of
# Managed Care Terms

In this section you'll find definitions for some of the terms you're likely to come across as you seek out and choose the best care and coverage for yourself. Some are described in more detail in the main text, and all are important to a complete understanding of HMOs and other managed care network plans.

**Ambulatory Care:** Health care that does not require a hospital admission for the patient—also called outpatient care—commonly provided in a doctor's office, clinic, or health center, but can also be provided in a hospital or "surgi-center."

**Anniversary Date:** The date on which a health plan's or insurer's contract with an employer or an individual subscriber is renewed each year. It is the date when premium costs and benefits are most likely to change. It may be preceded by an "open enrollment period," when employees have the option to switch health plans.

**Benefits or Benefit Package:** The health care services covered by a health plan or health insurance company, under the terms of its member contract. Terms of the contract also include any cost sharing required through copayments, deductibles, or coinsurance; limitations on the amount or length of coverage; and conditions such as the requirement to have care authorized in advance and delivered within the HMO network.

**Capitation:** A method of paying for medical services and health care on a per-person rather than a per-procedure basis. For instance, an HMO might pay a doctor a fixed amount per month for each HMO member he cares for, regardless of the type or amount of covered services the member requires. This creates a "budget" for all of the doctor's HMO patients. If the cost of their care is less than the budget, he keeps the difference; if it exceeds the budget, he takes a loss. Capitation contrasts with "fee-for-service" payment.

**Case Management:** A program or method that health plans and insurers use to coordinate the care of patients who have complex or expensive medical needs (or medical and nonmedical needs) to make sure they get the care they need in the most appropriate and cost-effective manner, and with the best possible outcomes. For instance, a case management team of doctors, nurses, and home-care workers might draw up and carry out a plan to help a car-crash victim move from acute hospital care to rehabilitation to care at home, with all of the needed services, medications, and therapies in each setting.

**Claim:** The documentation of a medical service that was provided to a covered patient by a doctor, hospital, laboratory, diagnostic service, or other medical professional. A claim is filed with the insurer by the provider or the patient to request payment (or reimbursement) for the service if the service was not prepaid.

**Clinician:** A term that is often used to describe all types of medical professionals who care for patients—doctors, nurses, physicians' assistants, therapists, etc.

**Coinsurance:** A cost-sharing arrangement typical to traditional health insurance, in which patients pay a portion of the cost of certain covered medical procedures, usually on a fixed percentage basis. For instance, patients might be required to pay 20 or 30 percent of the cost of their doctor's office fees or hospital charges for services they received. Usually coinsurance payments begin after an annual deductible is met.

**Community Rating:** A means of setting monthly health plan or insurance premium rates by estimating the cost of providing health care to the entire membership and dividing by the estimated number of members each month. With this method, each grouping within the entire membership population pays at the same rate. "Community rating by class" starts with the community rate and adjusts it up or down based on a given group's demographic (age and sex) makeup. "Adjusted community rating" starts with the community rate and, using a group's past use of medical services, adjusts it up or down based on an estimate of what the cost of providing health care to that group will be in the coming year. With "experience rating" the group's yearly premium rate is based on the actual cost of providing care to that specific group.

**Copayment:** A cost-sharing arrangement in which patients pay a fixed amount each time they receive certain covered services, no matter what the actual cost of the service is.

For instance, they may pay from $3 to $10 for any doctor's office visit, or $50 to $100 for any hospitalization.

**Deductible:** A cost-sharing arrangement typical to traditional health insurance in which patients must pay a fixed amount each year toward the cost of the covered services they receive before their insurer will start paying for coverage. For instance, a member might be responsible for paying the first $300 of her medical bills each year; after the deductible is met, the insurer would begin covering services at whatever level the contract calls for. Usually, deductibles are linked with coinsurance.

**Effective Date:** The date on which coverage under a health plan or insurance contract begins.

**Employer Contribution:** The amount of money an employer pays toward the health benefit plans of its employees. The employer may pay the same fixed number of dollars toward every plan it offers to its employees ("an equal-dollar contribution"); it may pay a fixed percentage of the premium for every plan offered ("equal-percentage contribution"); or it may adjust its contribution in other ways. The employee's portion of the health plan premium is typically paid through a payroll deduction.

**Enrollment Area:** The geographical area within which a health plan member must reside in order to be eligible for coverage. Most HMOs place a limit on the length of time members (except students) can live outside the enrollment area each year and still be covered.

**Federally Qualified:** An HMO that has met certain federal standards regarding financial soundness, quality assurance, member services, marketing, and provider contracts can be federally qualified. HMOs that are not federally qualified are still subject to federal and state regulations and requirements intended to protect consumers and providers and ensure quality of care.

**Fee-for-Service:** The method used by traditional health insurers to pay for medical services provided to their members: the medical provider charges a fee for each service, and the insurer pays all or a portion of that fee.

**Formulary:** A list of prescription drugs and their recommended doses, which have been selected by a health plan, insurer, or group of doctors as the best choices, in terms of effectiveness and value, among the many possible options for a given condition. Formulary drugs may be only recommended or they may be required as a condition of HMO prescription drug coverage (unless individual circumstances make a different drug a more appropriate choice for the patient). Formularies are used to manage both the cost and the quality of prescription drugs.

**Gatekeeper:** A term used to describe one role of a primary care doctor in an HMO or other managed care network that requires its members to have all of their care provided, arranged, or authorized by the members' primary care doctors, except in life-threatening emergencies or when temporarily "out of area."

**Health Screening:** A method used by some insurers and health plans to determine whether applicants are likely to create high medical costs, either because they are already sick or because they are likely to have a costly illness in the future. Health screening is used to detect preexisting medical conditions and to determine whether the applicant is at risk for illness because of factors like excessive weight or a past history of drug abuse.

**Inpatient:** Medical care that requires the patient to occupy a bed in a hospital. Not all hospital care is inpatient care; a patient can also receive "outpatient" care in a hospital's emergency room or ambulatory care center.

**Lock-in:** Refers to the requirement that members of an HMO or other managed network health plan must have all of their covered services provided, arranged, or authorized by the plan or its doctors, except in life-threatening emergencies or when members are temporarily "out of area." This contrasts with a "point-of-service" plan, which allows patients to receive covered services, without prior authorization but at a higher cost, outside the plan's network.

**Network/Participating Providers:** Used to describe the doctors, clinics, health centers, medical group practices, hospitals, and other providers that an HMO, PPO, or other managed care network plan has selected and contracted with to care for its members.

**Open Enrollment:** A period during which health plans or insurers accept new applicants for membership. Employers typically hold open enrollment periods each year to give their employees an opportunity to switch health plans if they want to (and if there is more than one option available).

**Opt-out:** The option available through some managed care network plans, such as point-of-service HMOs and preferred provider organizations, to choose to receive care from providers outside the plan's network, at a higher cost, and still be covered.

**Out of Area:** Beyond or outside of the geographical area served by an HMO or other managed network plan. When

HMO members are inside their HMO's service area, they must have their care provided, arranged, or authorized by their HMO or HMO doctor in order to get full coverage; when they are temporarily out of area, different coverage rules apply.

**Out-of-Pocket Costs:** The portion of the cost of health care and medical services that a person with health coverage is responsible for paying, usually through deductibles, coinsurance, or copayments.

**Preexisting Condition:** An illness or medical condition that an individual has before applying to a health plan or insurer for coverage. With some plans, individuals with certain preexisting conditions can be turned down for membership. Or they may be accepted for coverage, but with limitations on their coverage for preexisting conditions.

**Prepaid:** An arrangement in which those who provide care to a particular group of people are guaranteed payment in advance rather than having to seek payment from an insurer by filing claims for reimbursement for each service performed. HMOs are the most common type of prepaid health plans.

**Primary Care:** Preventive health care and routine medical care that is typically provided by a doctor trained in internal medicine, pediatrics, or family practice, or by a nurse, nurse practitioner, or physician's assistant, in a doctor's office, clinic, or health center. HMO members are encouraged or required to choose primary care doctors, who must provide, arrange, or authorize virtually all of the care they need.

**Provider:** A term often used to describe all types of health care professionals and facilities—doctors, nurses, physicians' assistants, hospitals, clinics, etc.

**Reasonable and Customary Charges or Fees:** An amount determined by an insurance company or HMO to be the appropriate amount to pay for a particular medical service because it is the average or commonly charged fee within a specific community. Insurers will often pay medical providers no more than reasonable and customary charges for covered services provided to their members.

**Referral:** A formal process by which a patient is authorized to receive care from a medical specialist or a hospital. HMOs usually require a referral from the member's primary care doctor or the HMO in order for specialty care to be covered.

**Risk:** An insurance term related to financial responsibility for medical care. A "high-risk" individual is someone who has a high likelihood of having a serious illness, because of past medical history, family history, or health-related behavior, such as smoking or alcohol abuse. "At risk" or "risk-bearing" means being responsible for the cost of care for a group of people. For instance, if an HMO pays a hospital a fixed amount of money per member to provide all of the care he or she needs, the hospital is "at risk" for that member. "Risk adjustment" means paying a health plan an extra amount if its members are, on average, sicker and more expensive to care for.

**Secondary Care:** A level of medical care between primary care and tertiary care, usually provided by medical specialists, and usually requiring a referral from an HMO member's primary care doctor.

**Self-Referral:** The ability for an HMO patient to refer himself or herself, under certain circumstances, for specialty medical care, without receiving a formal referral or prior authorization from the patient's HMO or primary care doctor.

**Self-Insured/Self-Funded:** An arrangement whereby employers pay directly for the health care services their employees need, rather than paying premiums to an insurance company or health plan for coverage. Some self-insured plans contract with HMOs or other managed care networks to provide all or most of their employees' health care. Services such as claims processing are usually furnished by a separate company, usually called a third-party administrator (TPA). This is referred to as an "administrative services only" (ASO) arrangement.

**Service Area:** The geographical area within which an HMO or other managed care network plan provides and arranges medical care for its members. This area is sometimes the same as the plan's enrollment area, but not always.

**Skimming:** A practice by which insurers or health plans try to avoid enrolling people whose medical care may be very expensive, including people who are elderly or who have a history of illness.

**Sole-Source Option:** A term meaning that an employer has chosen a single insurer or health plan to cover all of its employees. If the sole-source option is an HMO, it will usually offer both a standard lock-in plan and a point-of-service plan that allows members to choose to get care outside the HMO network, at a higher cost.

**Tertiary Care:** The upper level of medical care and services, usually provided in hospitals by highly trained "subspecialists" using the most advanced medical technology.

**Utilization:** The amount of medical services used by a given population, usually measured over a specific period of time or as an average related to the number of people in the population. For instance, an HMO's utilization rate for doctors' office visits might be five visits per member per year. Hospital utilization is often reported as the number of days in the hospital, on average, for each 1000 members of the group being measured (days/1000). In the interest of reducing costs, health plans and insurers try to reduce unnecessary or inappropriate utilization through "utilization management" or "utilization review."

**Waiting Period:** A period after the effective date of enrollment during which a new member of a health insurance plan is not covered for a preexisting medical condition.

# Resources

Following is a state-by-state list of the government agencies with primary responsibility for regulating HMOs. They should be able to provide you with information on which HMOs are offered in your part of the country, what kind of HMOs they are and how many members they have, whom they cover, what their average premiums are, and how you can contact them. They should also be able to alert you to any financial or other problems an HMO might be having.

Other sources of information, in addition to employers and the HMOs themselves, include:

►Local business groups: Chambers of Commerce, business coalitions, and associations have all become active in health care. Some states have business groups that focus entirely on health care. To find out if there is such a group in your state, check with your local Chamber of Commerce, or contact the Washington Business Group on Health, 777 North Capitol Street, NE, Suite 800, Washington, DC 20002.

►Federal government agencies: Ask directory assistance for the regional Health Care Financing Adminsitration office of the U.S. Department of Health and Human Services. Their Medicare and Medicaid divisions should be able to provide you with information about HMOs that enroll people in those categories.

## STATE HMO REGULATORS

Director of Insurance
P.O. Box 110805
333 Willoughby Avenue
9th Floor
Juneau, AK 99811
(907) 465-2515

Insurance Commissioner
135 South Union Street
Montgomery, AL 36130
(205) 269-3550
  and
Director, Life and Health
Department of Health
434 Monroe Street
Montgomery, AL 36130
(205) 613-5366

Insurance Commissioner
Suite 400
University Tower Building
1123 South University Avenue
Little Rock, AR 72204
(501) 686-2900

Insurance Commissioner
Office of the Governor
Pago Pago, American Samoa
  96799
(684) 633-4116

Director of Insurance
2910 North 44th Street
Suite 210
Phoenix, AZ 85018
(602) 912-8400

Insurance Commissioner
One City Centre Building
Suite 1120
770 L Street
Sacramento, CA 95814
(916) 445-5544
  and
Commissioner of Corporations
Department of Corporations
3700 Wilshire Boulevard
Suite 600
Los Angeles, CA 90010
(213) 736-3481

Commissioner of Insurance
1560 Broadway
Suite 850
Denver, CO 80202
(303) 894-7499

Insurance Commissioner
P.O. Box 816
Hartford, CT 06142
(203) 297-3857
and
Director, Life and Health
P.O. Box 816
Hartford, CT 06142
(203) 297-3857

Insurance Commissioner
441 4th Street, NW
8th Floor, North
Washington, DC 20001
(202) 727-7426

Insurance Commissioner
Rodney Building
841 Silver Lake Boulevard
Dover, DE 19901
(302) 739-4251
   and
Department of Public Health
Health Facilities, Licenses &
   Certification
3000 Newport Gap Pike
Wilmington, DE 19808
(302) 995-6674

Insurance Commissioner
State Capitol
Plaza Level Eleven
Tallahassee, FL 32399
(904) 922-3100

Insurance Commissioner
2 Martin L. King, Jr. Drive
Floyd Memorial Building
704 West Tower
Atlanta, GA 30334
(404) 656-2056

Insurance Commissioner
855 West Marine Drive
Agana, Guam 96910
(671) 477-5106

Insurance Commissioner
250 South King Street
Fifth Floor
Honolulu, HI 96813
(808) 586-2790

   and
Director
Department of Health
State Health Planning
   & Development
335 Merchant Street
Room 214 East
Honolulu, HI 96813
(808) 587-0788

Insurance Commissioner
Lucas State Office Building
Sixth Floor
Des Moines, IA 50319
(515) 281-5705
   and
Bureau Chief
Life and Health Department
Lucas State Office Building
Des Moines, IA 50319
(515) 281-4222

Insurance Director
700 West State Street
Third Floor
Boise, ID 83720
(208) 334-2250

Insurance Director
320 West Washington Street
Fourth Floor
Springfield, IL 62767
(217) 782-4515
   and
Director
Department of Public Health
535 West Jefferson
Room 500
Springfield, IL 62761
(217) 782-0382

Insurance Commissioner
311 West Washington Street
Suite 300
Indianapolis, IN 46204
(317) 232-2385

Insurance Commissioner
420 S.W. Ninth Street
Topeka, KS 66612
(913) 296-7801

Insurance Commissioner
215 West Main Street
Frankfort, KY 40601
(502) 564-3630

Insurance Commissioner
470 Atlantic Avenue
Sixth Floor
Boston, MA 02210
(617) 521-7301

Insurance Commissioner
501 St. Paul Place
Stanbalt Building
Seventh Floor, South
Baltimore, MD 21202
(410) 333-2521

Insurance Superintendent
State Office Building
State House, Station 34
Augusta, ME 04333
(207) 582-8707

Insurance Commissioner
611 West Ottawa Street
Second Floor, North
Lansing, MI 48933
(517) 373-9273

Insurance Commissioner
133 East 7th Street
St. Paul, MN 55101
(612) 296-6848
    and

Director of HMOs
Department of Health
121 East 17th Place
Suite 400
P.O. Box 64975
St. Paul, MN 55164
(612) 282-5600

Insurance Director
301 West High Street
Room 630
Jefferson City, MO 65101
(314) 751-126

Insurance Commissioner
1804 Walter Sillers Building
Jackson, MS 39205
(601) 359-3569
    and
Director
Health Department
421 West Pascagoula Street
Jackson, MS 39204
(601) 354-7300

Insurance Commissioner
126 North Sanders
Mitchell Building
Room 270
Helena, MT 59620
(406) 444-2040

Insurance Director
Terminal Building
941 'O' Street
Suite 400
Lincoln, NE 68508
(402) 471-2201

Insurance Commissioner
Dobbs Building
430 North Salisbury Street
Suite 3067
Raleigh, NC 27603
(919) 733-7349

Insurance Commissioner
600 East Boulevard
Bismark, ND 58505
(701) 224-2440

Insurance Commissioner
169 Manchester Street
Concord, NH 03301
(603) 271-2261

Insurance Commissioner
20 West State Street
CN 325
Trenton, NJ 08625
(609) 292-5363

Insurance Superintendent
P.O. Drawer 1269
Santa Fe, NM 87504
(505) 827-4500


Insurance Superintendent
State of New York
160 West Broadway
New York, NY 10013
(212) 602-0420

Insurance Commissioner
1665 Hot Springs Road
Carson City, NV 89716
(702) 687-4270

Insurance Director
2100 Stella Court
Columbus, OH 43215
(614) 644-2658

Insurance Commissioner
1901 North Walnut
Oklahoma City, OK 73152
(405) 521-2828
    and

Director of Health
Department of Health
1000 N.E. 10th Street
Oklahoma City, OK 73117
(405) 271-6868 ext. 263

Insurance Commissioner
21 Labor & Industries
    Building
Salem, OR 97310
(503) 378-4271

Insurance Commissioner
Strawberry Square
13th Floor
Harrisburg, PA 17120
(717) 787-5173
    and
Director
Department of Health
Bureau of Health Care
    Finance
Room 1026
Health & Welfare Building
Harrisburg, PA 17108
(717) 787-5193

Insurance Commissioner
Fernandez Juncos Station
1607 Ponce de Leon Avenue
Santurce, PR 00910
(809) 722-8686

Insurance Commissioner
233 Richmond Street
Suite 233
Providence, RI 02903
(401) 277-2223

Insurance Commissioner
1612 Marion Street
Columbia, SC 29202
(803) 737-6160

Insurance Director
State of South Dakota
500 East Capitol
Pierre, SD 57501
(605) 773-3563

Insurance Commissioner
Volunteer Plaza
5000 James Robertson
    Parkway
Nashville, TN 37243
(615) 741-2241

Insurance Commissioner
333 Guadalupe Street
P.O. Box 149104
Austin, TX 78714
(512) 463-6464
    and
Director
Health Department
1100 West 49th Street
Austin, TX 78756
(512) 322-4266

Insurance Commissioner
3110 State Office Building
Room 3110
Salt Lake City, UT 84114
(801) 538-3800

Insurance Commissioner
1300 East Main Street
Richmond, VA 23219
(804) 371-9694

Insurance Commissioner
Kongens Gade #18
St. Thomas, VI 00802
(809) 774-2991

Insurance Commissioner
89 Main Street
Drawer 20
Montpelier, VT 05620
(802) 828-3301

Insurance Commissioner
Insurance Building
P.O. Box 40255
Olympia, WA 98504
(206) 753-7301

Insurance Commissioner
State of Wisconsin
121 East Wilson
Madison, WI 53703
(608) 266-0102

Insurance Commissioner
2019 Washington Street, East
P.O. Box 50540
Charleston, WV 25305
(304) 558-3394

Insurance Commissioner
Herschler Building
122 West 25th Street
Cheyenne, WY 82002
(307) 777-7401

# Index